Living
and
Dying
at
Murray
Manor

Age Studies

Series Editor
Anne M. Wyatt-Brown, University of Florida

Living
and
Dying
at
Murray
Manor

JABER F. GUBRIUM

UNIVERSITY PRESS OF VIRGINIA

Charlottesville and London

The University Press of Virginia
Originally published in 1975 by St. Martin's Press, Inc.
© 1997 by the Rector and Visitors of the University of Virginia
All rights reserved
Expanded Paperback Edition
Printed in the United States of America

First published 1997
First University Press of Virginia edition published 1997

⊗ The paper used in this publication meets the minimum requirements of the
American National Standard for Information Sciences—Permanence of Paper for
Printed Library Materials, ANSI Z39.48-1984.

Library of Congress Cataloging-in-Publication Data

Gubrium, Jaber F.
    Living and dying at Murray Manor / Jaber F. Gubrium.—Expanded pbk. ed.
        p.   cm.—(Age studies)
    "With a new introduction."
    Includes bibliographical references and index.
    ISBN 0-8139-1777-8 (pbk.)
    1. Nursing home care.   2. Nursing homes—United States.
I. Title.   II. Series.
RA997.G77   1997
362.1'6—dc21   97-23621
                                                                          CIP

For Aline and Erika

Contents

Preface

Living and Dying at Murray Manor is not a survey of statistics about nursing homes; such information is available elsewhere.[1] Instead, it examines the social organization of care in a single nursing home that I have called Murray Manor.[2] My working question in preparing the book was, "How is care in a nursing home accomplished by those people who participate in its everyday life?" By "care" I mean whatever the participants consider to be part of life in a nursing home as distinguished from life in other places; by "people" I mean staff and clientele, as well as those who participate only fleetingly in life at Murray Manor, such as relatives, visiting physicians, and morticians. *Living and Dying at Murray Manor* documents the way in which the "work" of everyday life in a nursing home is accomplished: how the

[1] See, for example, chapter 25 of Matilda W. Riley and Anne Foner, *Aging and Society*, vol. 1 (New York: Russell Sage Foundation, 1968). Also consult the National Center for Health Statistics, *Vital and Health Statistics*, Series 12, Data from the Institutional Population Surveys (Washington, D.C.: U.S. Government Printing Office).

[2] Pseudonyms are used for people and places in the book.

participants negotiate their roles, goals, and needs; how they invoke their rights and duties; and how, in the end, Murray Manor emerges as an organized social entity.

To both the general public and to social scientists, life in a nursing home has come to mean decay, cruelty, and dehumanization. Such stereotyped images derive in part from journalistic exposés and local campaigns to "clean up those hovels." [3] Although it is true that some aspects of life in nursing homes match these stereotypes, life at Murray Manor is filled wih intimate social ties, the celebration of small accomplishments, agonizing losses, boredom, conspiracies, anger, pride, humiliation, trust, love, hope, despair—in short, all the complexities that occur when a group of people spend their daily lives together.

Nursing homes vary in a number of ways. They differ, of course, in the quality of the care provided. They may provide residential care, medical care, or a combination of both. They may be proprietary homes operated under private commercial licenses, nonprofit homes operated under voluntary auspices, or government homes run by local, state, or federal agencies. They vary considerably in the number of beds and occupants. Murray Manor is a nonprofit, church-related home offering both residential and medical care. According to data collected in the National Health Survey in April–June 1963,[4] Murray Manor, with 360 beds, is considered a large nursing home. The occupancy rate at Murray Manor at the time I conducted most of my field work (1973) was about 36 percent, and it has grown steadily to a current rate of about 60 percent.

I spent several months at Murray Manor, in 1973, as a participant-observer. In the course of my study I took many roles, ranging from doing the rather menial work called "toileting" by people there to serving as a gerontologist at staff meetings. I at-

[3] In the last ten years, the nursing home industry has had its share of public criticism. See Mary Adelaide Mendelson, *Tender Loving Greed* (New York: Knopf, 1974); Claire Townsend, *Old Age: The Last Segregation* (New York: Grossman, 1971); and U.S. Senate Subcommittee on Long-Term Care, *Conditions and Problems in the Nation's Nursing Homes*, Parts 1–7, 89th Cong., 1st sess., 1965.

[4] National Center for Health Statistics, "Institutions for the Aged and Chronically Ill," *Vital and Health Statistics*, PHS Pub. No. 100, Series 12, No. 1, Public Health Service (Washington, D.C.: U.S. Government Printing Office, 1965).

tempted to spend sufficient time in the setting to establish trust, to interact with as many people as possible, and to observe the varied facets of life at Murray Manor in their natural states.

Field work takes time—a great deal of it. I thank the Committee on Research of Marquette University for its generous Faculty Fellowship to study Murray Manor.

In a study such as this, expressing appreciation to one's subjects is always a problem. One owes so much to them, but can only celebrate them anonymously. For their openness, warmth, and willingness to show me their lives and talk to me of their "troubles," I am indeed grateful to the staff members and clients of Murray Manor.

For other kinds of help, I thank the following people: Jenny Delp, for painstakingly transcribing tapes of interviews and conversations; Margret Ksander, for comparing notes on "her" nursing home; Dave Buckholdt and Paule Verdet, for reading and commenting on the original manuscript; Shelly Buckholdt, Sharron Johns, and Sharon Skinner, for typing the manuscript; and my wife, Suzanne, who supported the project in many ways and kept our two children sufficiently occupied so that I could write.

I am indebted to Arthur Strimling of St. Martin's Press. He showed interest in my idea at first sight and encouraged me to realize it. The fine copyediting of Susan Rothstein is much appreciated, as well as Anita Morse's able and expeditious management of the whole project at St. Martin's.

Introduction

It has been twenty-five years since I conducted the fieldwork that led to the publication of *Living and Dying at Murray Manor.* For many months in 1973, I participated in and observed the daily round of life and the work of caregiving at a nursing home I eventually called "Murray Manor." The research opened my eyes to a sad world, but also one that revealed the complicated meanings of living and dying in an institution. My aim in writing the book was to bring those complicated meanings to light, to document that from the participants' perspectives. As in the classic Japanese film *Rashomon,* which cinematically compares how different points of view reveal events, I used the concept of "worlds" to emphasize how the nursing home, while a single organization, was virtually different worlds for the administrative staff ("top staff"), front-line workers ("floor staff"), and the clientele.

A DEVELOPING RESEARCH GENRE

At the time, there was very little written of sociological significance about the nursing home. There were the usual newspaper accounts and exposés of poor quality care and patient abuse, which of course alerted the public to the nursing home as a social problem. There also were various and sundry government reports and statistical analyses that provided an "accountant's" kind of view of the condition of long-term care. In comparison, the research literature on the sociology of the nursing home was meager. Few social researchers had taken the time to document how caregiving was actually done and received. One of the only available studies was a comparative analysis of a hospital and two nursing homes by anthropologist Jules Henry (1963), who gave a quite negative view of the homes, calling one of them "Hell's Vestibule" because of its filth and neglect. A few studies by sociologists were just appearing, such as Elizabeth Gustafson's (1972) article on the moral career of the nursing home patient and Charles Stannard's (1973) article on the social organization of abuse in the nursing home. May Sarton's (1973) fictional account of elderly nursing home resident Caro Spencer's experience in a facility Sarton called "Twin Elms" was forthcoming.

Since then, an exciting area of social research called nursing home ethnography has emerged (see Henderson and Vesperi 1995). If the area highlights the complex worlds of caregiving, it also provides perspectives on the everyday meanings of those worlds. For example, anthropologist Renée Rose Shield's (1988) participant observation in a northeastern U.S. nursing home focused on the problem of liminality for residents, that is, the transition experience of going from an accustomed role to a new institutional one. Shield presents to us the everyday meanings of adjusting to living in a context that uneasily combines the cultural codes of both hospital and home. In another ethnography, anthropologist Joel Savishinsky (1991) offers a lively account of life in an upstate New York nursing home and shows how storytelling by both residents and staff contributes to the developing meaning of the surroundings, memories, illness, and loss. Sociologist Timothy Diamond (1992), who himself was trained as a nursing assistant, makes use of his acquired skills to show us, from the perspective of the working staff member, how aides and orderlies manage to offer care while under the combined pressures of home, family, and low wages. His is also a trenchant discussion of the local consequences of corporate profit-making. Anthropologist Nancy Foner (1994) focuses on the strains and daily cross-pressures facing nurse's aides, considering in particular how the culture of aides' work offers a set of meanings for helping them to adapt to their jobs. Taken together, these and other studies in this genre expand our understanding of what it means to live, work, and die in a long-term care institution.

WHAT'S CHANGED SINCE THE EARLY 1970S?

Several noteworthy changes in long-term care have come about since the early 1970s when the Murray Manor fieldwork was conducted. One change has been how the nursing home as an institution fits into the overall continuum of care, that spectrum of institutions and other settings, from the hospital to the home, that treat and otherwise care for people. If the idea of a continuum of care has been subjected to critical analysis (see Gubrium 1991), the nursing home is still often figured to be a caregiving institution that lies somewhere between the acute care hospital and the family home. While the nursing home doesn't provide surgical procedures and other highly technical medical interventions, nor feature the comforts of home in terms of being the location of extensive personal belongings and the individual control of daily life scheduling, it does offer medical and nursing cares and usually does try to present these in surroundings that seem "like home."

Today's nursing home is closer to the acute care hospital end of the continuum than it was in the 1970s. Nursing home care today is more specialized (Mor, Banaszak-Holl, and Zinn 1995). There may be formally designated subacute care units for postacute hospital care, requiring physician supervision and skilled nursing services combined with physiological monitoring on a continuous basis. Increasingly, nursing homes are forming special care units, or SCUs, for Alzheimer's and other dementia patients. These units are usually locked and do not as much provide skilled nursing care as custodial services and monitoring. There also may be special units for rehabilitation, in which patients regularly receive physical and occupational therapy such as stroke and orthopedic rehabilitation. While still rare, some nursing homes even offer hospice care with units set aside for the terminally ill, usually untreatable cancers.

Murray Manor did not have special care units of any kind. SCUs were rare, if nonexistent, in those days. Instead, like most nursing homes, the Manor divided its services into skilled and intermediate nursing care and personal care. The first floor was a personal care unit, which furnished residents services similar to those offered in what are now called "assisted living" facilities. Referred to as "residents," not "patients," those who resided on the Manor's first floor, sometimes together in the same room as husband and wife, received help with dressing, bathing, and medication monitoring as needed. All were required to be ambulatory and cognitively alert. The Manor's other floors offered various levels of nursing care, the case-mix of "patients" ranging from those with various kinds of chronic illnesses and those in need of physical rehabilitation to the demented (often diagnosed with organic brain syndromes), vegetative, and comatose. (Because I needed a general term of reference for both residents and patients in writing the book, I called them all the "clientele.") Still, even though SCUs did not exist at the Manor, room assignments tended to concentrate patients with special care problems into particular areas for ease of monitoring. For example, it was not uncommon for dementia patients to be assigned rooms close to the nurse's station, so that the floor staff could "keep an eye" on their whereabouts.

Some say that market forces will move the nursing facility even closer to the acute care hospital in the future (Morris 1995). In the early 1980s, Medicare's prospective payment system for hospitals, based on diagnosis-related groups, or DRGs, provided flat payments to hospitals for the treatment of various groups of diagnoses. In contrast to a retrospective payment system, where hospitals could charge for each service rendered, they were now paid a fixed amount by Medicare on the basis of diagnosis. As a result, hospitals began to discharge their patients "quicker and sicker." One outcome was that nursing homes, to which hospitals often discharge their patients when they aren't sent home, began to admit sicker patients than ever (Estes, Swan, and Associates 1993). Combined with the increasing specialization of care in nursing homes, the result will be that the distinction between these facilities and hospitals in the future will be even more blurred.

Another market force contributing to change is the rapid development of assisted living facilities and home health services. Assisted living facilities make available the kind of personal care offered by the Manor in the early 1970s, except that assisted living facilities are usually freestanding. They furnish apartmentlike accommodations, congregate meal plans, and help with activities of daily living (see Golant 1997). The growth of the home health industry means that patients who formerly might have had to be cared for in a nursing facility can now be cared for at home, in some cases virtually bringing the hospital home (Arras 1995). These developments have affected the nursing home in that its case-mix is now likely to include fewer of those who can be housed in assisted living or cared for at home.

It is important not to overestimate these kinds of change. While market forces do operate to shift the nursing facility more toward the hospital end and less toward the home end of the continuum, nursing homes still are not hospitals. The average length of stay in the nursing home remains significantly longer than that of the hospital. The many long-stay residents who live in nursing facilities for over six months and often much longer, are presented the poignant experiential issue of making a new home, as much as they receive nursing cares. Typical hospital stays of a few days obviate the issue, not challenging patients with the trials and dilemmas of permanent relocation. The nursing home case-mix continues to include mentally alert and ambulatory patients in need of nursing cares for a variety of chronic and postacute needs. Nursing homes are not becoming facilities predominantly serving the demented, even while some have such SCUs and the pool of eligible residents is living longer and thus more likely to have dementia symptoms. Still, dementia symptoms are not Alzheimer's disease. While the nursing home may be becoming more rationalized in its service categories, the case-mix is still in many ways what it always was, with the exception perhaps of the distinctly personal care once offered by nursing facilities like Murray Manor.

Changes in addition to those along the continuum of care are noteworthy. As one would expect, the cost of nursing home care, like the cost of health care in general, has risen significantly since the early 1970s. *Living and Dying at Murray Manor* lists the daily cost of various levels of care for the Manor at the time of the field-work (p. 8). Costs ranged from $15 per day for a semi-private room on the first floor for what is listed as residential care, to $39 per day for a private room on other floors for what was then categorized as maximum (skilled) nursing care. Today, the average per diem rate for skilled nursing home care in a private room is $111 (Assisted Living Federation of America 1996). In comparison, the average per diem rate for subacute care is $250. Given these figures, it would have cost approximately $14,000 per year to be cared for at the maximum level in a private room at Murray Manor in the early 1970s. The current annual cost for a comparable level of care would average about $40,500. Of course, then as now, the figures don't reflect who pays for this care, which can vary depending on whether residents themselves pay (private pay) or the cost is covered by other sources, most commonly Medicaid.

Another noteworthy change is the shifting racial and ethnic composition of both nursing home clientele and the nursing staff, especially the floor staff. No longer does the nursing home cater to a relatively homogeneous clientele. Residents are decreasingly likely to be white and mainly middle-class. Increasing numbers of African Americans, Latinos, and other minorities are being cared for in nursing homes, as their primary family caregivers are more and more employed outside the home. Rightly or wrongly, the belief that minorities prefer to care for their elders at home is being overshadowed by the fact that the traditional minority home caregiver is gradually disappearing into the job market. The result is a growing minority nursing home clientele that doesn't orient to nonfamilial care in the same way their white counterparts do (Belgrave, Wykle, and Choi 1993; Wallace 1990). The racial and ethnic composition of the nursing staff, still mainly female, also has become more heterogeneous. Whereas the typical nurse's aide in the early 1970s was either white or African American, now she is more likely to work alongside aides with other racial and ethnic backgrounds (Maas, Buckwalter, and Specht 1996). As commentators have pointed out, this staff/clientele heterogeneity can be the breeding ground for misunderstandings and conflict (Snyder 1982; Tellis-Nayak and Tellis-Nayak 1989).

But here again it is important not to overestimate the change. In the early 1970s, it was not unusual in having African-American nurse's aides on staff. While most of the patients and residents at Murray Manor were white, some had distinct ethnic backgrounds. If interpersonal racial and ethnic relations between floor staff and clientele were not the focus of my fieldwork, I nonetheless observed occasional disagreements between staff and clientele that centered on such differences. The white clientele could resent being cared for by African Americans and, in turn, the African-American aides could resent the haughty way they were treated by some white patients and especially a few residents. While I don't mean to suggest that these and other racial and ethnic differences weren't important in staff/clientele relations at the Manor, they were part of the way differences of any kind generate annoyances and disagreements. What has changed in this regard is not that such difference-linked problems are new in nursing homes but, rather, that they have broadened. Thus, what might have been annoyances and disagreements stemming from racial differences in the 1970s now include those centered on both race and ethnicity such as might arise not only between a white resident and a black aide but also between an elderly African-American patient and an Asian or white aide.

Another change worth mentioning is the emergence of quality of care assessment systems for nursing facilities. This is not to say that there was no concern during the early 1970s with the quality of care at Murray Manor. As is evident in the chapter entitled "Top Staff and Its World," the administrative staff aimed to make Murray Manor the "best nursing home in the country" and the facility was known to be one of the finest in the area. There were regularly scheduled patient care conferences, in which long-term and short-terms goals were set for caregiving, which were periodically reviewed or revised as needed. Patients and residents were continually monitored and caregiving and clientele conditions systematically charted by the floor staff. The recent development of the so-called Resident Assessment Instrument (RAI), part of nursing home reform legislation during the 1980s, did not so much lead to new forms of monitoring as it expanded and rationalized existing activity nationwide. Whether this in itself has led to better quality care from the client's point of view is open to question (Gubrium 1993). There is no doubt that the RAI provides a basis for measuring quality of care as understood by service provider consultants (see Murphy, Morris, Fries, and Zimmerman 1995). Still, overall, whether it is the result of increased monitoring of this kind, new state and federal regulations, clientele advocacy, or a climate of patient rights, the quality of care and the quality of life for clientele are in general better today than they were years ago (Vladeck and Feuerberg 1995).

WHAT HASN'T CHANGED SINCE THE EARLY 1970S?

In considering what hasn't changed since the early 1970s, let's return to the concept of "worlds," which I mentioned at the start. The concept signifies wholeness and borders. As it applies to people, a world can refer to all that a person or group knows or experiences. We sometimes say, for example, that a particular person's world is limited to his family and work, suggesting that anything outside these realms of experience is irrelevant to him. Such a person organizes his affairs around work and family, thinks of his past in these terms, and plans for his future accordingly. The concept also applies to groups. For instance, a group of friends might be so "into themselves," as it's sometimes put, that they appear to be living in their own little world. By this, we mean that they organize their lives in relation to each other, not outsiders, and define their individual identities in terms of being group members.

It's an important concept because it informs us that, as we attempt to understand people's lives, we might well consider that there are experiential borders to what they think, feel, and do. To say that a group lives in its own little world informs us that we might consider what it is about their sense of commonality—the wholeness of their own little world—that guides individual actions. We might ask how group members organize their sentiments and make decisions in response to this world. Now, I don't mean to suggest that worlds determine what their members think and feel or how outsiders respond to them. People, after all, do have their own senses of these worlds and, in that regard, can decide to criticize them, act out of character, or otherwise challenge their *working* borders. I deliberately emphasize the term *working* because it connotes wholeness and borders that only pose practical limits.

What's more, worlds are always subject to collision with other worlds, to borrow from the title of science fiction writer H. G. Wells's book *When Worlds Collide*. A group of friends who live in their own little world not only have constructed a border that experientially circumscribes and organizes their own relations and sentiments but the border, for better or worse, also shields them from other worlds, from other individuals and groups who have similarly organized their lives. As long as borders are intact and worlds remain relatively separate from each other, their respective members conduct their lives and interact in terms of their own shared understandings, in relation to how they expect the whole to inform its membership and their relationships. Of course, members of a world are never totally at peace with each other; there are, after all, individual differences, which produce variations in what is shared.

One way to think about how worlds affect us is that they make experience reasonable. To be part of a little world, for example, is to take for granted that what one and others do in the context of that world makes sense to them. Members of a world don't have to offer excuses to each other for what they think, feel, and do, or otherwise account for their actions. As members, they think, act, and express their sentiments in relation to each other in quite understandable terms. Indeed, the taken-for-grantedness may operate so that little or no attention at all is paid to what is or isn't reasonable, life simply going on for members as if nothing else mattered.

This is the way I eventually came to view the worlds attendant to living, working, and dying at Murray Manor. When I first began my fieldwork, I had a quite stereotypic sense of what nursing home life was like, most notably the generally poor quality of long-term care so often communicated in the media. When I mentioned what I was studying, the immediate response was usually "Oh, those awful places you read about." There were more personal reactions, too, such as the adult daughter who told me flatly, "I would never put Mother in one of those." Before I started my observations, I had never been in a nursing home and knew no one who lived or worked in one. There was no reason to think that, as an organization, Murray Manor or any other nursing facilities were more complicated than the image the public held of them. The nursing home was an organization that left much to be desired as a health care setting, certainly more than a hospital or a home.

At the same time, my natural skepticism took hold. Some say that this character trait always stands a fieldworker in good stead, encouraging him or her to see for themselves and not be duped by received wisdom or public understandings. It led me to wonder if the nursing home simply was Hell's Vestibule? Suppose I chose to study the very best nursing facility I could find. Would I just find an organization that didn't leave quite as much to be desired as a health care setting? My wonder and these questions were informed by what I reminded myself Erving Goffman (1961) had written years earlier about his own fieldwork at St. Elizabeth's, a psychiatric hospital, which is worth quoting in full: "My immediate objective in doing fieldwork at St. Elizabeth's was to try to learn about the world of the hospital inmate, as this world is subjectively experienced by him. . . . It was then and still is my belief that any group of persons—prisoners, primitives, pilots, or patients—develop a life of their own that becomes meaningful, reasonable, and normal once you get close to it, and that a good way to learn about any of these worlds is to submit oneself in the company of the members to the daily round of petty contingencies to which they are subject" (pp. ix–x).

It suggested that I take a look for myself, to get a firsthand view.

I had already contacted several facilities because I had originally planned to do a survey of the quality of care in nursing homes from the point of view of the clientele. (This was eventually set aside and not taken up again until twenty years later. See Gubrium 1993.) One nursing home administrator, whose name I fictionalized as the Mr. Filstead of *Living and Dying at Murray Manor,* showed the kind of interest in my questions that I later realized was an ethnographer's dream. Filstead was research-oriented and wanted to help improve the quality of care in nursing homes. He told me that he admired my desire to get a firsthand view of things and not be satisfied with the one-dimensional approach to nursing facilities that was being bandied about in the media. So he invited me to "take a look" for myself and the fieldwork began.

As I interacted with the staff and the clientele, it wasn't too long before I started to feel Goffman's objective tapping me on the shoulder. While Murray Manor was the best nursing home in the region, if not the country, and did nonetheless leave something to be desired as a health care facility, it was far from simply being *an* organization or just *a* nursing home. I started to see that the daily lives and work of administrators, floor staff, residents, and patients offered remarkably different perspectives on the meaning of care and caregiving. It occurred to me that a single nursing home, when considered from the points of view of its distinct categories of participant, might be several different organizations in practice. I used the term *world* to convey the difference because it suggested something separate and distinct from the outside and yet whole and reasonable from within. Regular references by the floor staff to "them," meaning the administrative staff, conveyed a sense of being outside of important channels of decision-making affecting their work. Comments such as "we" know what we want, meaning what patients desire as opposed to what staff considers is best for "them," signaled a shared reasonableness among equals that outsiders couldn't, or perhaps wouldn't, understand.

My sense was that administrators ("top staff"), as well intentioned as I actually found them to be, worked in a separate world from the floor staff. What the top staff saw as good and efficient caregiving, floor staff could consider "just getting the job done." The residents and patients, too, lived in their respective worlds, which separated them in terms of what they took for granted as reasonable expectations from the floor staff. What a resident felt was time well spent chatting with a friendly nurse's aide could, from the aide's point of view, be time away from other duties. The aide, after all, was not only providing care but also doing a job, themes that Diamond (1992) and Foner (1994) would elaborate much later.

The indigenous reasonableness of these separate worlds was not only secured by perspective but by what I eventually called "place." By and large, top staff conducted their daily affairs in their offices and in meetings. Those places helped to keep their world separate and distinct from other worlds, its knowledge and sense of what is reasonable intact and unchallenged. Floor staff, especially nurse's aides, spent most of their work lives on patient and resident floors, caring for and mingling with clientele and each other. Rarely did they attend top staff meetings, nor did they otherwise much enter into top staff's world. The clientele, too, carried on life in their own places, in their own rooms, the dining areas, lounges, and other locations on their floors. The clientele were further subdivided into informal friendship circles, cliques, and mutually supportive dyads, each with their own little worlds and customary places of interaction. In contrast to top staff, floor staff and clientele regularly came into contact with each other. As a result, their worlds were more likely to collide than top and floor staff's, causing the usual kinds of related incidents and complaints. As long as worlds operated in separate places, these troubles were at a minimum. But they often didn't operate that way, and I figured that the way place affected worlds was a useful means of understanding what nursing homes were like as settings for living, working, and dying.

So, to answer the question of what hasn't changed in nursing homes since the early 1970s, I can say that they remain health care settings internally differentiated into the worlds they have always been. They still have top and floor staffs and there still are clientele. They are, in effect, still *socially* differentiated and organized. Their qualities as places to give care, to live, and to die are still responsive to these differentiations. While in the 1970s they could have been much better places to work, live, and die, which they now seem to be as Vladeck and Feuerberg (1995) point out, they remain organized into their separate worlds. In that regard, work and life within them can be improved only up to a point, which is the point at which the nursing home combines living, working, and dying into a single going concern. Renée Shield (1988) has noted that the nature of the beast called the nursing home combines the cultural codes of hospital and home, thus reaping a distinct horizon for caregiving and good care. Simple as it might seem, my own view is that in addition to this, the nursing home, Murray Manor included, as a configuration of worlds and places, continues for better or worse to make living, working, and dying there as reasonable as it can possibly be. That is the continuing significance of the fieldwork done years ago.

REFERENCES

Arras, John D. (ed.). 1995. *Bringing the Hospital Home: Ethical and Social Implications of High-Tech Home Care.* Baltimore: Johns Hopkins University Press.

Assisted Living Federation of America. 1996. *An Overview of the Assisted Living Industry.* Fairfax, Virginia.

Belgrave, Linda L., May L. Wykle, and J. M. Choi. 1993. "Health, Double Jeopardy, and Culture: The Use of Institutionalization by African-Americans." *Gerontologist* 33: 379–85.

Diamond, Timothy. 1992. *Making Gray Gold: Narratives of Nursing Home Care.* Chicago: University of Chicago Press.

Estes, Carroll L., James H. Swan, and Associates. 1993. *The Long Term Care Crisis.* Newbury Park, CA: Sage.

Foner, Nancy. 1994. *The Caregiving Dilemma: Work in an American Nursing Home.* Berkeley: University of California Press.

Goffman, Erving. 1961. *Asylums.* Garden City, NY: Doubleday.

Golant, Stephen. 1997. "The Promise of Assisted Living as a Shelter and Care Alternative for Frail American Elders: A Cautionary Essay." In *Aging, Autonomy, and Architecture: Advances in Assisted Living,* edited by Benyamin Schwarz and Ruth Brent. Baltimore: Johns Hopkins University Press.

Gubrium, Jaber F. 1991. *The Mosaic of Care: Frail Elderly and Their Families in the Real World.* New York: Springer.

Gubrium, Jaber F. 1993. *Speaking of Life: Horizons of Meaning for Nursing Home Residents.* Hawthorne, NY: Aldine de Gruyter.

Gustafson, Elisabeth. 1972. "Dying: The Career of the Nursing Home Patient." *Journal of Health and Social Behavior* 13: 226–35.

Henderson, J. Neil, and Maria Vesperi (eds.). 1995. *The Culture of Long-Term Care: Nursing Home Ethnography.* Westport, CT: Bergin & Garvey.

Henry, Jules. 1963. *Culture against Man.* New York: Random House.

Maas, Meridean, Kathleen Buckwalter, and Janet Specht. 1996. "Nursing Staff and Quality of Care in Nursing Homes." Pp. 361–425 in *Nursing Staff in Hospitals and Nursing Homes,* edited by Gooloo

S. Wunderlich, Frank A. Sloan, and Carolyne K. Davis. Washington, DC: National Academy Press.

Mor, Vincent, Jane Banaszak-Holl, and Jacqueline Zinn. 1995. "The Trend toward Specialization in Nursing Care Facilities." *Generations* 19: 24–29.

Morris, Robert. 1995. "The Evolution of the Nursing Home as an Intermediary Institution. *Generations* 19: 57–61.

Murphy Katharine M., John N. Morris, Brant E. Fries, and David R. Zimmerman. 1995. "The Resident Assessment Instrument: Implications for Quality, Reimbursement, and Research." *Generations* 19: 43–46.

Sarton, May. 1973. *As We Are Now.* New York: Norton.

Savishinsky, Joel S. 1991. *The Ends of Time: Life and Work in a Nursing Home.* New York: Bergin & Garvey.

Shield, Renée Rose. 1988. *Uneasy Endings: Daily Life in an American Nursing Home.* Ithaca, NY: Cornell University Press.

Snyder, P. 1982. "Creating Culturally Supportive Environments in Long Term Care Institutions." *Journal of Long Term Care Administration* 10: 19–28.

Stannard, Charles I. 1973. "Old Folks and Dirty Work: The Social Conditions for Patient Abuse in a Nursing Home." *Social Problems* 20: 329–42.

Tellis-Nayak, V., and M. Tellis-Nayak. 1989. "Quality of Care and the Burden of Two Cultures: When the World of the Nurse's Aide Enters the World of the Nursing Home." *Gerontologist* 33: 307–13.

Vladeck, Bruce C., and Marvin Feuerberg. 1995. "Unloving Care Revisited." *Generations* 19: 9–13.

Wallace, Steven P. 1990. "Race versus Class in the Health Care of African-American Elderly." *Social Problems* 37: 517–34.

Gainesville, Florida
April 1997

Living
and
Dying
at
Murray
Manor

1 | The Setting

THE MEANING OF PLACE

In their everyday routines, people come to accept different places as having certain meanings. They maintain such located meanings by, in effect, talking about the "right things in the right places." The meanings of places and their props are not intrinsic to them, however. In a very mundane sense, people in places make them meaningful, although this task usually goes unnoticed. Each person tacitly believes that his work has been preceded by the work of others who had specific place expectations. Furthermore, he knows that his work is presently contingent on still others with similar expectations. This knowledge of the place expectations of others affects talk and gesture in the ongoing interaction among participants in any place. Through unwitting routines, people make locations meaningful and tend to maintain these meanings as practical solutions to getting on with the affairs of living together for some time in some place.

These meanings are not settled, once and for all, when they have been routinized. A person may choose to be "difficult" and risk having to negotiate his deviance with others who, at least for the moment, have accepted the meaning of the place. Or one of the perennially loose ends of place such as missing props may suggest to all persons in that place that they remake its meaning. Or the meaning of certain places may virtually run out or run over in the course of time, urging their participants to ask, "What gives here?" It is on such occasions of instability that the precarious meaning of place becomes most obvious.

THE PARTICIPANTS

People who make part or all of their everyday lives at Murray Manor may be divided into two general categories: staff and clientele, with further meaningful distinctions existing within each group.

Staff

Staff consists of all employees in the various departments of the nursing home, plus the home's administrator and medical director. These departments are accounting, social services, nursing, maintenance, housekeeping, dietary, central supply, recreation, pastoral care, and occupational therapy (OT). Those departments that staff believes deal directly with clientele care in terms of professional therapeutics are often referred to as the various disciplines; they include social services, nursing, dietary, recreation, occupational therapy, and pastoral care. All personnel in these disciplines, from the least to the most prestigious, are considered to be involved in rehabilitating or maintaining clientele. Employees in departments not called disciplines are not expected to take a therapeutic attitude toward clientele; their work involves running the home, not "running" its inhabitants.

The difference between conceiving of work as running the home and therapeutics influences the formal attitude of staff members toward clientele. Although all staff members, in practice, deal with clientele as fellow members at Murray Manor, differences occur in how they go on record as, or publicly profess to be, working with them. Therapeutic staff frames its official references to and reports of work with clientele in the language of rehabilitation, referring to itself as "working on" Murray Manor's clientele. It considers clientele first as patients and second as rational, self-interested human beings. Nontherapeutic staff, on the other hand, has no formal obligation to describe its work in terms of clientele rehabilitation or maintenance.

The sizes of the various departments differ considerably. All but the nursing department have from one to ten members. The nursing department employs about 65 people distributed unequally over three shifts: "days" (7 A.M. to 3:30 P.M.); "P.M.S" (3 P.M to 11:30 P.M.); and "nights" (11 P.M. to 7:30 A.M.). The total size of the nursing staff varies; its erratic but persistent turnover is due to the mobility of nursing personnel in an employees' labor market.

Members of the staff also differ in the amount of time they work on the floors with clientele.[1] Some, mainly nursing personnel, spend all or most of their time there. Nursing personnel on the floor consists of the charge nurse on each floor, who is usually a registered nurse (RN); supporting licensed practical nurses (LPNs); and varying numbers of nurses' aides. In addition to the nursing personnel, one or two housekeeping aides are on the floors for most of their workday, doing such tasks as vacuuming rooms, washing toilets and basins, dusting furniture, and disinfecting urine- or stool-stained carpeting. I shall refer to the nursing and housekeeping employees as the floor staff.

The activities of the floor nursing staff fall into three categories. First, the charge nurse supervises other nursing personnel on her unit, delegates work assignments and patient loads, and performs a variety of floor-related administrative tasks such as taking telephone orders from physicians and ordering drugs from the pharmacy. Supporting LPNs may be delegated some of this administrative work, and occasionally they act as charge nurses. Second, RNs and LPNs administer patient treatments and distribute medications. Third, aides tend to bed-and-body work on clientele, such as helping them to void, eat, turn in bed, dress, bathe, and smoke.

The members of the Manor staff who spend little or no time on the floors, and who usually are found in their offices or in a variety of conferences, are the administrator, medical director, and the heads of the various departments. Those that administer work that deals directly with clientele care are the administrator, medical director, social worker, director and assistant director of nursing, in-service director, activity director, occupational

---

[1] Floors are also called "units" and sometimes "wards." The administration prefers not to use the latter term, however, since Murray Manor is considered to be a home, not a hospital.

therapist, chaplain, and dietitian. I shall refer to these members of the administrative staff as the top staff.

These distinctions between various departments and staff positions are meaningful mostly to the staff itself and only to some clientele. In their relations with each other, staff members often invoke the relative prestige of their status in the disciplines when they feel it is to their advantage. However, they ignore status when it is obvious that doing otherwise would hamper their attempts to gain information or to elicit support for a policy position they are taking. For example, in trying to convince the administrator that a certain procedure for handling clientele belongings is more efficient than another one, the social worker at Murray Manor cites her training in social relations to support her case that she knows "what's best for these people." The head housekeeper, preferring the alternate procedure, has no recourse to invoking such expertise. In another context, the social worker gossips with the housekeeper, who unwittingly provides information about the relations between two allegedly troublesome patients on the third floor. The social worker is obviously exasperated and confesses, "I just don't know what the hell we're going to do with those two." The housekeeper makes an off-the-cuff remark about what she'd do if "I were in your shoes." Later, the social worker presents this suggestion to the administrator, ignoring its source and embellishing it with an appropriate psychological rationale.

To clientele, the ability to make distinctions in talk and deed between various staff members depends on their felt needs and relative physical mobility. Those ambulatory clientele who are dissatisfied with some aspect of their lives in the home readily seek the "top brass" or the "head guy in this place." For instance, it is common for grumbling clientele who are irritated with what they consider to be "lousy, cold food" to collect one or two other able persons and "go down to that kitchen and complain about the poor treatment we're getting in this place." Such dissatisfied persons make it their business to know "who's the boss of who" in order to use such knowledge in influencing staff members. They may threaten "to report" certain employees if "they don't straighten out what's going on here." They know of and make distinctions between members of the floor staff and generally are aware of who is the charge nurse on each shift and who are nurses' aides.

On the other hand, clientele who are mostly confined to their beds or wheelchairs tend to have a narrower conception of differences among staff members. To many of these clientele, all those who work on the floors, including the housekeeping aides, are simply "nurses." This lack of distinction, in turn, affects their demands on the staff. They become irritated and impatient with any "nurse" who refuses to do for them what another nurse will readily perform. "Nurses" who state that they cannot fulfill certain requests (e.g., nurses' aides may not officially dispense medications, and housekeeping aides do not do bed-and-body work) or who fetch an RN or LPN to attend to these requests are likely to be defined by the physically limited clientele as inconsiderate, lazy, or "too busy with themselves to do some little thing for you." Members of the floor staff are aware of this lack of clientele knowledge of the formal organization of employees at the Manor, and when it is in their interest and the place is appropriate, they use it to their own advantage. Knowledgeable clientele, on the other hand, keep staff "on their toes." As any aide soon realizes, and one aide reports,

> You know who's got their cookies and who doesn't. Mrs. Sealy [patient]—now if you don't treat her just so-so, she'll report you to Filstead [administrator] or Miss Timmons [director of nursing]. She's [Sealy] got her marbles and won't take the same stuff that the others [some other clientele] do. Some of the others don't know who in hell's who. You can relax with them. They'll yell, but that's as far as it goes.

Clientele

Clientele at Murray Manor are categorized in various ways. One classification, based on the state's definition of levels of skilled nursing care, is meaningful only to the top staff. The distinction is made between residential, minimum, moderate, and maximum nursing care; this is based on the level of skilled nursing care a patient needs. This classification is important to the top staff for two reasons: first, staff/patient ratios required by the State Nursing Home Code depend on the level of skilled care given to clientele; second, state and federal remuneration for nursing home care varies by the level provided.

Clientele are also categorized by the floor on which they

reside. Persons housed on the first floor are, officially, only in need of personal domiciliary services and are called *residents.* Residents should be ambulatory and not require skilled nursing care. Persons who reside on the third and fourth floors are considered to be in need of various levels of skilled nursing care and are referred to as *patients.* Some are ambulatory and some are bedridden. Together, residents and patients constitute the clientele of the nursing home. Other floors at Murray Manor currently are unoccupied.

This classification is meaningful to both staff and clientele. Top staff uses it in its work with floor staff and in its infrequent interactions with clientele. Floor staff and clientele use it almost exclusively in their relations. In talking about patients as distinct from residents, the floor or floors occupied by these respective classes are used as a reference. It is common for residents to speak of "the people upstairs," or "those people on the third floor." Likewise, patients talk about the "first floor," or "down there."

In practice, the fact that clientele physically reside on either the first, third, or fourth floor does not necessarily mean that they are always considered and treated as either residents or patients. Clientele and staff construct these clientele distinctions as needed, such a construction being contingent on persons' immediate interests, their felt needs, time, and place. For example, when a particular resident "got to be a bit goofy," another one stated, "He should be put upstairs. He really doesn't belong down here. Down here, everyone can take care of themselves. He bothers everyone." Or take Gus Marsh, also a resident, who became angry with the "ten-year-old stuff" that Don Staats was "handing out to some of the old maids":

> Yes, there's one man. He's on a vacation this week. His son got 'em. He gives everybody trouble. He's loud and he's filthy-talking. They call him Don. He come to me and I don't even answer him. He wants to make conversation. And the women—he calls 'em sons-of-bitches too— loud as hell and stuff. Two or three times, the nurse will come up and quiet him down and take him to his room and stuff. I don't think he belongs here. He belongs on a different floor or a different institution or something. A man talkin' like that to a bunch of women and stuff, that's why.

When a staff member is disgusted with a resident, the staff member may make subtle comments such as: "That's not the kind of thing we do down here, Mr. Goldman. You don't see other residents acting like that, do you?" This reminder of the precarious nature of clientele classifications serves as a way to control a resident's behavior.

A blind patient who had become a fast friend of several residents is the center of a persistent campaign by the residents to have her moved to the first floor because "Blanche has more marbles than most do even on this floor [first]. She can get around just as good as the rest of us. She's no patient! They should put Goldman or Staats upstairs in Blanche's place." With no top staff on the scene, Sharon Sewell (third-floor RN) corroborates the residents' sentiments about Blanche:

> She's a good self-help. They [top staff] asked me if she could go downstairs and I said, "Yes." I think they're keeping her up here because they get more money out of her up here. Also, she does need minimal supervision but we could train her up here and get her ready for the first floor. She just doesn't belong up here. They've got us in a bind. We were training her on how to make her bed, but we can't do it and tell her it's because it's training for downstairs since they've given us no guarantee that she's going downstairs.

Patients, residents, and staff make other distinctions among various members of the clientele. These distinctions are not tied to place as definitively as those between residents and patients. Residents and patients are sometimes classified by staff, as well as each other, as senile or not senile; having all their marbles, some of their marbles, or none at all; alert or not alert; confused or not confused; in reality or out of reality; and oriented or disoriented. These labels, like others, are convenient for people to use in dealing with each other in various situations.

There is a daily fluctuation in clientele census at Murray Manor. Currently, there are about 130 persons residing in the home, one-third of whom are residents and the rest patients. The census fluctuates with admissions, live discharges, and deaths. The number of patients or residents on a floor varies as transfers are made from one floor to another. The nursing home can accommodate 360 patients and residents on 6 floors (60 beds per floor). This number of beds is slowly being filled.

The average age of patients and residents is just over eighty years. Although Murray Manor formally refers to itself as a geriatric care faciltiy, it occasionally admits a patient who is fairly young. The clearest instance is the admission of a twenty-seven-year-old female terminal diabetic who is given approximately four to six months to live and has been classified as in need of extensive skilled nursing care. The only other patient under sixty years of age admitted to Murray Manor was a woman in her forties who has since been discharged. Residents, on the other hand, are all aged.

As might be expected in any population of the aged, females outnumber males by about four to one at Murray Manor. The average age for females (80.5 years) was slightly higher than for males (80.1 years) in one of the months in which data were gathered. Most clientele are admitted from hospitals (about 65 percent). Some come from home (about 25 percent) or from other nursing homes (about 10 percent). Discharges vary in the same proportions; most are to hospitals, next to homes, and a few to other nursing homes.

Although Murray Manor is a nonprofit, church-related institution, no religious restrictions are placed on admissions.[2] About 60 percent of its clientele are Catholic, 38 percent Protestant, and 2 percent Jewish.

Two-thirds of the clientele pay for their care personally, others are supported mainly by funds provided by Title 19 of the Social Security Act (Medicaid). Room rates per day, based on the level of skilled nursing care, are:

	SEMI-PRIVATE	PRIVATE
Residential care	$15	$25
Minimum care	20	35
Moderate care	22	37
Maximum care	24	39

Currently, only 6 out of 130 patients occupy private rooms.

[2] Its board of directors is comprised of seven Catholic nuns representing three orders plus three lay members. With the exception of the chaplain, all members of the top staff are lay people and more are Protestant than Catholic. All but two or three members of the floor staff are lay people.

KINDS OF PLACES

Murray Manor as a physical setting has many places; that is, locations in which people do things that are meaningful, reasonable, and taken for granted because of where the people are and who is with them. Two meaningful dimensions of place are whether it is public or private, and how this status changes over time. Some places tend to be public most of the time, whereas others tend to remain private. However, the stability of either is a product of the routineness with which members *treat* places as public or private.

A public place is a location that a member makes no effort through talk or gesture to claim as his or her own. A private place is a location the member considers his or her own. It has boundaries that admit only the member's presence and claim to its privileges. The primary distinction between public and private places is whether a person has been defined as the only claimant of a location's privileges. Even though a place may be considered public as long as a single claimant to its privileges has not been made known, this does not mean that the members of a public place are unlimited. There is always a relevant public (acceptable members) of a place who are taken for granted as legitimate occupants of its premises, for the time being. Relevant publics change in time, sometimes routinely and sometimes fleetingly.

The dimension of timing is such a central and yet perverse feature of the meaning of place that one has to come to terms with it analytically in order to describe how place works. One way to do this is to divide places into those that are, more or less, routinely public or private at certain times and those whose status is continually negotiated.

Although a place may be considered private by a member, this does not mean that no one else is on its premises. A member's claim of exclusive rights to the privileges of a place may or may not involve the tacit assumption that other people be present to make good such a claim. In some cases, a member of a private place may need others to assist him in its use but not to indulge in its use themselves. In such a case, other people become part of the privileges of private place. For instance, an aide may enter a patient's room to help him with his toilet and still maintain the privacy of the place. But entering without such a purpose would be considered a violation of privacy.

The Physical Layout

Murray Manor is a large nursing home, with 6 floors, and 30 rooms on each floor. Every room has accommodations for 2 persons, although anyone may contract for its private use. In addition to living facilities, the building has a wing used for a variety of clientele and administrative services.

Figures 1, 2 and 3 show the physical arrangement of the basement, first, and third floors. In the basement are located a variety of house services. The first floor is for residents, with the main lobby on the same level. The third and fourth floors house patients and have virtually the same layout.

The Basement. The offices and service areas of dietary and departments not considered disciplines are located in the basement. Patients' and residents' laundry is done here. The housekeeper's office is located here, as are central supply and maintenance. The north wing of the basement contains the employees' lounge, with staff lockers and lavatories to one side. A general-purpose classroom located near the lounge is used for such things as in-service training and conferences.

The basement has one important external feature. A service ramp running along the east side of the south wing of the building descends from the street level to the maintenance area. It is used for the delivery of such things as foodstuffs and medical supplies and the collection of garbage and bodies.

The First Floor. The first floor is the site of the main public entrance to the building, the lobby, the receptionist's counter, and the offices of the social service department and the administrator. The building entrance faces north, opposite to where the service ramp is located. The entrance contains a foyer, which is mostly a public place, although occasionally it is treated as private. It is enclosed on two sides by glass doors, one set facing the outside, the other facing the lobby. One wall of the foyer is glass, which also looks onto the lobby. The foyer has usually one and sometimes two chairs in it, against the back wall. Anyone sitting in it has an expansive view of two busy areas of the nursing home: the entrance walk and visitors' parking area, and the lobby.

All visitors, most employees, and service personnel such as physicians, clergy, and physical therapists enter the building through the main entrance. They pass through the lobby and often make some gesture to or ask a question of the receptionist

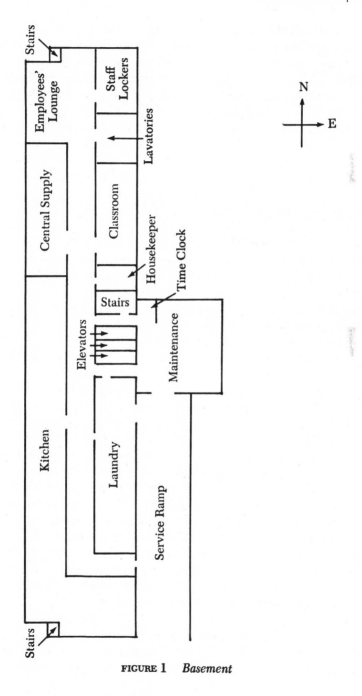

FIGURE 1   *Basement*

before proceeding to their destinations. Clientele, mostly residents, also pass through the lobby on their way outdoors. If they leave the immediate premises of the nursing home, they are supposed to "check out" with the receptionist. The social worker and administrator, whose offices are located along the east wall of the lobby are often seen chatting as they pass through the lobby on their way to other offices or locations. There are three elevators; the main one opens onto the lobby as well as onto the first-floor hallway, and the other two, with only one door, are often used as service elevators. All in all, anyone who is frequently present in this area and is watching and listening will see and hear a great deal of and about certain participants in everyday life at Murray Manor.

In addition, the lobby has two places where persons may sit and, of course, watch and listen to events. In the lobby proper, the public waiting area, an arrangement of sofas and chairs next to the elevator, centers on a table with a variety of magazines on it. The receptionist bids visitors to sit there while they are waiting for a member of the administrative staff. On the other side of the foyer's single glass wall is a small, physically separate side lobby which has four armchairs. Like the foyer, it provides a good view of the entrance and the lobby proper. It is officially considered a public place, but it also has its definite private moments and private negotiations.

The residential area of the first floor is composed of a long hallway (260 feet) divided in half by the nurses' station, a curved counter about four feet high that faces the elevators. On the first floor, its height is not behaviorally significant; however, on the third and fourth floors, staff may use it to hide from wheelchair patients whom they wish to avoid. To the immediate left and right of the station are fire doors that are kept open, but that close automatically during fire drills. Residents' rooms line either side of the hallway. At both ends are open areas without doors. The area at the north end of the hallway is a lounge containing two or three groupings of armchairs, several small tables, and a television set. The area at the south end serves as a dining room for residents as well as a lounge. It does not have a television. Next to the nurses' station, in what was once a resident's room, there is a gift shop. Here clientele display and sell their wares. Supplying the shop with items is one way of passing time at Murray Manor.

Behind the nurses' station are two small cubicles called "med rooms." They contain medical supplies, paper products, and medications as well as a sink. It is amusing to members of the floor staff that the med room is also the place where residents' alcoholic beverages are stored.[3] Their amusement has two facets. At first encounter it is surprising to find that, as one LPN declared, "a veritable bar hits you in the puss just when you expect to find pills and cotton wadding." Second, it is continually ironic to some members of the floor staff that "people this age are still interested in booze and sex."

Midway between the nurses' station and each lounge, there is a bathroom. Each has two tubs and a shower stall, plus a toilet. The bathrooms, like all other clientele places, have no locks. Because many people have easy physical access to the bathrooms but most residents consider bathing a private affair, the extent to which the bathroms are private or public places has been the source of no small number of "causes" at the Manor.

In addition to the bathrooms and the single toilet in each resident's and patient's room, each floor has a visitors' toilet and a staff toilet. The visitors' toilet is next to the elevator; the staff toilet is next to one of the med rooms behind the nurse's station. There are, then, 34 toilets on each floor. Some patients or residents take advantage of the one nearest to them in time of need; others honor what they consider private places. Depending on the choice, there may be composure or momentary chaos on the floor.

The building has three stairways, one at each end of the hallway and one near the elevators. Officially, these are fire escapes. Staff members in a hurry use them instead of waiting for elevators. Residents and patients use them occasionally, too—sometimes to go to the basement and sometimes to escape what they consider their nursing home imprisonment without being detected by the nursing staff. Each stairway has an exit to the outside on the first floor.

The Grounds and Environs. All clientele presumably have access to the Manor's grounds. In practice, the personal as well as administrative difficulties that must be overcome in order to

---

[3] All medications and alcoholic beverages are dispensed only by physician's order. This includes patent medicines such as drugstore aspirin, laxatives, and salves.

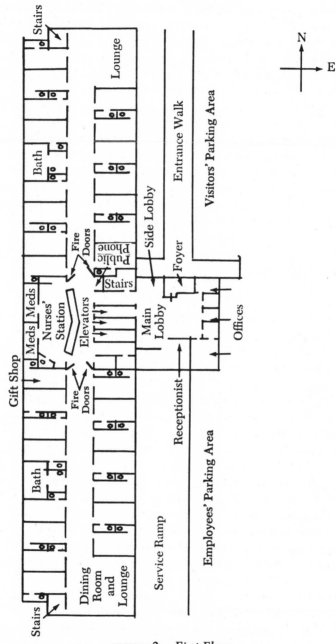

FIGURE 2   *First Floor*

go outside vary from residents to patients. Patients not only have a more difficult time physically managing themselves out-of-doors because of bodily incapacities, but floor staff often requires that they be accompanied there either by an aide, another patient, or a resident. Who the person is accompanying the patient will depend on floor contingencies ranging from shortage of help on specific days to shifting staff assessments of the patient's self-reliance.

The grounds consist of four areas in which patients, residents, or staff may be found, singly or interacting together. Along the entrance walk, considerable activity is found in warm, fair weather. On its periphery, there are usually five or six multi-colored park benches. One faces north and is adjacent to the main entrance; the others face east and line the walkway. The one is at times a more private place than the others, for it may be claimed by certain "ladies" on the first floor.

A second area is the lawn and flower garden along the east side of the building. Besides Bill Munger, the Manor's maintenance man, a few residents spend some of their day tending to certain claimed chores here.

A third area is found along the west side of the building; it is a strip of grass, about 15 feet wide, that has little or no daily use by anyone except by an occasional person who crosses it in going around the building or taking a shortcut between the streets bordering the home on the north and south. On rare occasions, it is the scene of outdoor ceremonials such as a cook-out for clientele.

The parking lots on the east side of the building, the short drive in front of the main entrance, and the service ramp at the southeast corner constitute a fourth area of the grounds. Visitors park in the north lot. Employees park toward the rear of the building along the east side. Activities in these areas serve as clues, for patients and residents, to who is in the home at the moment and to past or impending events, such as a death having occurred or the clientele services to be offered on that particular day.

The lots, short drive, and ramp are not equally visible from each patient's or resident's room. Those with rooms on the west side of the home cannot observe the activity in these areas from their windows. Those on the northeast have a view of the visitors' parking lot and drive; and those on the southeast look onto the service ramp and employees' parking area from their rooms. This differential access to the grounds where daily activity related to the Manor occurs makes for some specialization by patients and residents in spreading newsworthy events. Of course, anyone presumably would have access to a panoramic view of events on the grounds by looking out of the windows of either lounge. This does not typically occur because lounges, like clientele rooms, have differing social claimants and differential physical accessibility to patients and residents.

A few places outside the building, although not part of the Manor's grounds, may nonetheless be considered part of its physical setting. First, the building is located at the center of a city block, occupying a complete cross-section of it. In fair weather, clientele may be found walking around the block or half of it, sometimes alone but usually in company. Second, bordering streets on the north and south are major thoroughfares. Watching and considering the traffic that passes there is an important pastime for clientele. Third, there is a snack shop on the next block that it is frequented by a few residents. And fourth, about three blocks to the north is a small shopping center, and those residents who can "make it there on foot" boast of their accomplishment.

The Other Floors. The third and fourth floors at Murray Manor house patients and are similar in layout to the first, with a few exceptions. The beauty and barber shop is located on the third floor, and any residents or patients wishing their hair set or cut must come there to have it done. To residents, this is risky business since they all have heard and some "know" about the "poor souls" and "nuts" that "you might run into up there." The physical therapist, who comes to the Manor from a local rehabilitation center at certain scheduled times, uses the rear of the fourth-floor dining area. On the third and fourth floors, the dining rooms are located above what is the lobby on first. Both are uncarpeted in contrast to the residents' dining room. They are the scene of eating, smoking, bingo games, incontinence, and just plain sitting around.

Two other floors have places where patients and residents may be found at various times of the day. On the fifth floor, the recreation and occupational therapy departments are located in the east wing (the area above the third- and fourth-floor dining rooms). This is the location of such events as arm and hand exer-

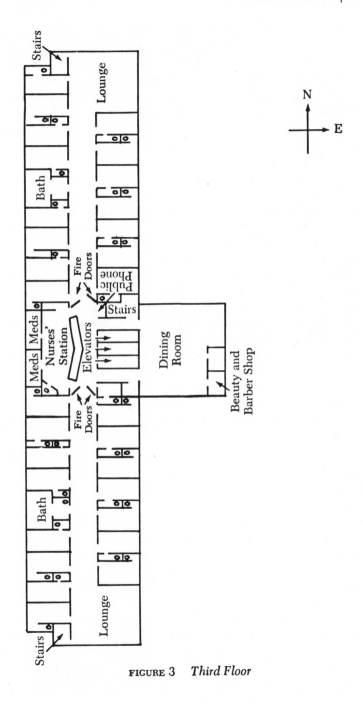

FIGURE 3   *Third Floor*

cises, birthday parties, sewing, and cooking. As in the beauty and barber shop on the third floor, and the physical therapy (PT) area on the fourth, patients and residents mingle with each other here—often inadvertently, sometimes quite uneasily.

The chapel is located in the south lounge area on the second floor. It is used for both Catholic and Protestant services, one on Sunday morning and the other on Sunday evening. In addition, it is used by Catholics for saying the rosary on weekday afternoons. Both patients and residents attend these events. In contrast to other places at Murray Manor where residents have contacts with patients, residents tend to be most cordial, indulgent, and helpful to patients going to, during, and coming from religious services. The meaning of this place is sanctity. It is rarely violated, not even, strangely enough, by the "real loonies."

The second floor is also the location of the administrative nurses' offices, which are located in its east wing. Doors leading to this area are always closed. Rarely are residents, let alone patients, to be found here. However, it is the site of considerable top staff activity. When top staff deals with assembled floor staff, such meetings usually occur in the basement. When top staff confers privately on what it believes to be policy matters or simply to gossip as a group, it often does so in a small conference room in this area or in one of the administrative nurses' offices.

Clientele Rooms. The resident's or patient's room is the final component of the physical setting of Murray Manor. Its private character is at times negotiable. (A typical room is shown in Figure 4.) All rooms are the same size, and each has a single window. The bed next to the window is called "bed 2," and the question of who occupies this place may be problematic, since to many patients and residents it is the more desirable place in the room. All rooms have a small, closet-sized cubicle with a door to one side, which has a toilet and buzzer cord to the nurses' station. Each bed also has a cord on the wall, usually at its head. There is a single large closet with no provisions for separate identification of clientele clothing. This is also problematic and leads to many crises over privacy. A single sink is located in the room proper, next to the door of the toilet room.

The particular location of a room along the hallway is important to some patients and residents. Some prefer to have sunny rooms; for this, a southeast location is preferable. Many know that "what's going on outside" is more accessible from a room with a window that faces east. Also, on each floor, being located as far as possible from patients or residents who are considered undesirables is preferred. Comments referring to certain ends of the hallway in a negative way are not uncommon. Blanche Holden, a blind patient with a room located on the far south wing of the third floor, put it this way:

> Well, you know. Most of them are older. And they're senile, some of them. Most of them are. There's only a few of us here that are not. Those two men—Stanley Semke and Mr. Cooper and Mr. . . . What's his name now? Those are the only few right now. Those on the other side. Oh my! Oh my! They're not so good. They're all . . . ach . . . I said already. If I have to live with them much longer, I'll get senile from hearing them talk.

The persons who make such remarks may overlook the fact that they have friends in the same area of the hallway where they've located undesirables.

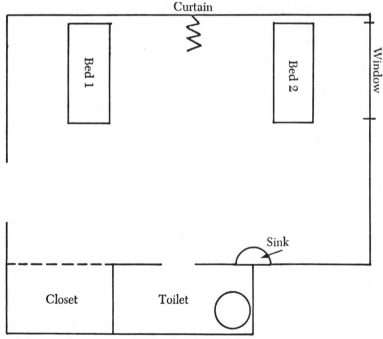

FIGURE 4   *Clientele Room*

Room furnishings vary considerably. Although most patients and residents have identical hospital beds and nightstands, some have added chairs and dressers of their own to their rooms. Most rooms have such personal effects as pictures, radios, television sets, lamps, bedspreads, plants, and bookcases. Many residents and a few patients have private telephones in their rooms.

Room decor is a source of pride to many clientele. Upon first entering a room, one is usually shown the whole gamut of belongings that its occupant has added to its basic furnishings. This is true of both men and women. All point with pride to the cards or small gifts they had received from children or other relatives on the last holiday.

If any photographs are displayed in the room, they are invariably brought to one's attention with such typical explanations as: "That's my daughter." "I have ten grandchildren. Here's their picture." "See my nephew. Isn't he good-looking?" However, upon meeting the people who appear in such photographs, they are usually considerably older than portrayed.

Although no clientele rooms on any floor can be locked, they all have doors that can be closed. On the first floor, when residents are not in their rooms or consider themselves indisposed, their doors are usually shut. Walking into someone's room without knocking or in the temporary absence of its occupant is considered, at best, rude and presumptuous. Although some third- and fourth-floor patients respond similarly, most do not.

PUBLIC PLACES

The Basement

The Manor's basement is officially public to all staff. In practice, however, at certain times specific places are public only to the floor staff. When members of the floor staff become aware of top staff's presence, they redefine areas in such a way that all personnel on the premises become "good employees." Upon redefinition, the content of talk about work and patients is conscientious and service-oriented. Top staff believes that any good employee at Murray Manor is dedicated, interested in "total patient care," and part of a "quality service team." In the company of top staff, floor staff supports this belief.

The employees' time clock is located in the maintenance area. At shift change, hourly employees gather around it to check in and out. There is much milling about and some gossiping. It is taken for granted that at shift change the time clock area is employee territory. No one expects the administrator or other members of the top staff to appear, and they hardly ever do.

Murray Manor's administrator, Mr. Filstead, and its director of nursing, Miss Timmons, believe the area to be an ideal location for the communication of new procedures or policy decisions to employees. These communications, called directives, are posted next to the clock on the wall or on bulletin boards. They conceive the place to be one where each *individual* employee punches in or out and *each* checks carefully for posted announcements. Employees, on the other hand, often arrive and depart en masse, are usually in the hurried business of punching in or out, and do not notice memos when they are posted there. There is rarely any commentary about the memos.

When a so-called directive is noticed by someone, loud and sarcastic comments often are made that intimate that, as one aide said flatly, "Filstead doesn't know what the hell's going on upstairs. I'll just do what I have to do with the patients and tell 'em [top staff] what they want to hear." Everyone agrees, nods, or shrugs their shoulders. They all know that top staff is rarely on the floors.

The employees' lounge is another public place in the basement. Most members of the floor staff and some members of the top staff take their breaks here. Many also eat their lunches and dinners in the area. The lounge is the location of a great deal of talk about such things as "difficult" patients, patient romances, lazy co-employees, complaining relatives, meddlesome administrators, and allegedly "stupid" policies, as well as other topics not related to work in the nursing home. Because top as well as floor staff members are both present at times, everyone is constantly wary of "who's around."

Depending on who is present in the lounge, who departs, or who enters, its public character may shift from a place where "you can let it all hang out," to one where talk is supportive of top staff's image of the "team." Some members of the top staff are not considered by floor staff to be, as its members say, "as uptight as others." For example, the in-service director, although an administrative nurse, is believed to be someone who "understands the problems that you have with these patients." When she enters the lounge, talk among floor staff does not shift dramatically in tone or content. The entrance of other members of the top staff, especially the administrator, will, however, alter the public character of the lounge altogether. Upon seeing top staff enter, aides make a variety of gestures to each other, signifying their presence. For example, those who notice the administrator may widen their eyes, slyly stiffen, and subtly blink to one another in his direction.

The classroom is a "good employee's" place. It is public to floor staff on two occasions. In-service training classes are held here, and floor staff is asked to attend sessions on a variety of topics ranging from fire drill procedure to the care of terminal patients. It is also the location of what are called patient care conferences (PCCs), meetings held to "staff," or review, the medical care and/or behavior of certain patients and residents. Occasionally, select members of the floor staff are asked to attend PCCs to provide top staff with, as the medical director often states, "the benefit of your experienced expertise."

In the classroom, members of the floor staff are attentive to and indulgent of their superiors. They make it obvious that they are "part of the team," as the administrator frequently describes them. At PCCs, if top staff diagnose a certain patient's behavior as disoriented and confused, invited aides publicly concur; if top staff prescribes more TLC (tender loving care) for a certain patient, aides agree. At the next staffing of the same patient, aides are likely to report that what was prescribed was or was not effective in altering that particular patient's behavior, depending on how they interpret the sentiments of top staff.

The basement at Murray Manor is not routinely public to clientele. When clientele appear there, their presence is negotiated. How negotiation proceeds and ends depends on how the parties involved define each other, as well as on how clientele account for their presence on the floor.[4]

Whether or not clientele accounts are treated as possible justifications or excuses for their presence in the basement is affected by staff definitions of clientele competence. Accounts offered by clientele who are considered by the staff to be completely senile are not honored, no matter how rationally presented. An allegedly

---

[4] For an analytic treatment of the sociology of accounts, see Marvin B. Scott and Stanford M. Lyman, "Accounts," *American Sociological Review* 33 (1968): 46–62.

disoriented patient who says that he wants to "see someone in charge because I've got a complaint about what I have to pay here" is humored, indulged, and coaxed back to his room. The basement is not public to him.

Take Sal Zenda, a patient from the third floor. On one occasion, Sal decided that he wasn't "getting my money's worth," as he says, and intended to do something about it by complaining to someone "in charge." He took the elevator to the basement where there are a few administrative offices. Sal entered the housekeeper's office and told her that he wanted to talk to someone in charge about the services he was getting. After a few polite exchanges, she asked him to sit down while she called upstairs to see "if the man in charge is in." While he waited, the housekeeper called the third floor and informed the charge nurse that Sal was in the basement. The nurse and two aides appeared in the basement two minutes later.

Now, it is important to note here that Sal is considered very disoriented by the staff. As an aide mentioned, "You really can't take anything he says seriously." Being disoriented officially means that his talk is believed to have no connection with his actions and to provide no clues to the causes of his behavior. The talk of such people is ignored by floor staff. No matter what Sal says, staff "knows better."

To ignore a disoriented person's talk as a way of managing him is not the same as to ignore it altogether. The staff member provides the appearance that the patient's or resident's talk is being taken into account while directing interaction toward a different end. This means that when Sal asks to see the "boss," the housekeeper says "yes" and then calls someone else. It means that aides tell Sal that "the man in charge is not in right now," and that they'll take him upstairs where he can wait for him—as they lead him back onto the elevator to the third floor. It also means that when Sal reappears on the third floor, he is told to wait in his room and that he'll be notified "as soon as the boss gets in." Through coordinated subterfuge, the sanctity of place is momentarily restored.

Although no personal accounts offered by "disoriented" patients justify their presence in the basement, there is one situation in which an account does legitimate the presence of such a patient here. This is an account offered by someone else for the patient.

Mike Helmut, a fourth-floor patient, rarely goes anywhere in the Manor except to walk up and down the hallway near his room. Although he's ambulatory, staff considers him to be otherwise incapable of self-care or rational decision-making. To one aide (Sharon Menske), who often attends to Mike, he is charming and pleasant. She has adopted him as a patient of "special interest to me." He knows this and so does the staff on the floor.

Sharon occasionally takes Mike down to the employees' lounge for a soda. When it is time for her break, she readies him, and they proceed down the elevator to the lounge—together. If there should happen to be other staff members present in the lounge, Sharon mentions to Mike in a clear and distinct voice that is obviously meant for everyone in the room, "Now, let's have a soda and sit down for a while, Mike." This signifies to those present that she, after all, is in control of the situation, and it accounts for Mike's presence there. Without it, those in the lounge would whisk him away to his proper place on the fourth floor.

Anyone considered senile who appears unaccompanied in any place in or out of the nursing home other than on the floor where he resides is defined by the staff as "escaping." No matter what such a person says, it is taken for granted that "that's not where he belongs." For such patients who are accompanied by a staff member but who are momentarily left alone, this is somewhat problematic at times. They have been known to be "properly" whisked away by other vigilant staff members, to a temporarily absent aide's dismay. On such occasions, a slapstick series of events may follow that does not always rectify matters to everyones' satisfaction. To one aide, a patient's been found; to another, he's "escaped"; and to the patient, his change of scene has been rudely cut short. His objections, of course, go unheeded as he's warned to "stay put."

Patients and residents considered by the staff to be alert receive a different treatment in staff places. As long as they can provide a legitimate account for their presence in such places, the places are public to them. The range of acceptable accounts, however, is usually fairly narrow. In the basement at Murray Manor I have known only a few kinds of accounts to be judged legitimate by the staff. When residents and patients are asked why they are "down here," they occasionally say that they have a specific request or complaint to make to the kitchen, laundry, or housekeeping service. Sometimes clientele are in the company of relatives for whom they are obviously providing a tour of the home. Both accounts are acceptable. Also, they may state that they made a mistake with the elevator and it let them off on the wrong floor. Staff is likely to be more skeptical of this excuse than the others since, from the elevators, the basement appears so different from all the other floors.

The First Floor

Patient and resident floors at Murray Manor differ in the extent to which they are generally public places. The residential area on the first floor is less public to all clientele than are the third and fourth floors. In the first-floor residential area, it is routine to see only a few walking residents and perhaps one or two staff members in the hallway, and one or two people sitting in the north and south lounges. The mood is quiet, unrushed, and cordial. Anyone in this area usually is fully dressed, except at certain commonly prescribed hours such as breakfast time and late in the evening. Most doors to residents' rooms are closed. Anyone found in the north lounge usually resides on the north wing. The same is true of the south lounge. The atmosphere is one of genteel living.

Three residents describe the first floor in the following ways:

> I don't know too much about 'em [patients]. I just don't. We're on our floor and they're on their's. It's a good way of classifying them. The ones down here can take care of themselves. And I never go up on third floor. It's just that we don't belong up there. It's noisier up there. That's not for me.
>
> ──────
>
> . . . half of 'em [patients] don't know how to find their way back [to their rooms]. That's third- and fourth-floor stuff. These on this floor are more or less sane people but they're handicapped. Oh, one or two get a little radical. They get a little loud on certain subjects, just like in any group. Once they get their point over or something, then it's over with. They're a pretty normal group; just they have their peculiarities.
>
> ──────
>
> We're all residents down here—all in our right minds— and know what we're doing and where we're going. And, most everybody on this floor has the privilege to go and come as they feel like it. We're not locked up. I can go any time I want and any place I want. But, you get up-

stairs, you'll find out. It's quite different. Then you will truly see the inside of the institution. There's some pitiful cases up there. Very pitiful.

A number of events violate the public areas of the first floor. Except for a select few, who "everyone down here knows don't belong upstairs," patients are not considered to belong "down heie." Residents continuously make a very clear distinction between their floor and its lifestyle and "those people upstairs." Whenever one of the patients "escapes," as they say, "you never know what they'll do down here." Residents are very concerned about maintaining the quiet decorum of their floor. Gus Marsh, a resident, relates two cases where "it's just a plain damn fact that this place is not for them."

> The nurses say that's a rough place up there. Then, there are one or two of 'em that sneak out and you have to catch them. They don't like the place. Sal, especially. He's an ex-boxer and his wife is a nurse at Mason. How he gets out—he gets out. First thing you know, you see him down the street. The nurses come down lookin' for him. One of them runs this way and one of them runs this way. "See Sal?" "Yeah, he went out the door." You got to call him Sal and talk nice. A week ago Saturday, he was really mad. He was down here and wanted to see the district attorney. That's the kind of cases you get. Then, we had a woman. She took off. One of the girls that carts her around—she just swiped that girl one. Knocked her clear on her fanny on the grass. It took 'em ten minutes to get her in that elevator. You wouldn't dare to come close to her. She'd smack you one right in the gut. Finally, they caught her arms and gave her a little pill, I guess. Calm them down and stuff. Oh, what a racket she made.

Both first-floor lounges have their proper publics. No official rule states that certain residents must use one rather than the other; in practice, however, residents usually frequent the lounge closest to their rooms. Each lounge is believed to have its room-specific personnel.

The practical public character of each lounge makes it possible to locate many residents on the floor when they are not in their rooms but are somewhere on the premises. Asked where a certain resident is to be found when not "at home," another one is likely to answer, "try that lounge up there." The belief about who belongs in which lounge also is used as a rationale for dissuading someone considered undesirable from frequenting a specific lounge. For example, Dorothy Porath, whose room is in the south wing, has been known to watch television in the north lounge and fall asleep on the couch, "letting it run until late at night." She's been told by several women with rooms near the lounge to "go to the other end, Dorothy, where you belong." Don Staats, who also resides in the south wing and who is considered to have a "dirty mouth," often sits in the north lounge with a friend who has a room near it. Whenever these women run into him there they scoff at his presence and snidely tell him that he has his "own place down at the other end." They add, "Why do you want to bother everyone down here?" Don typically spits back, "Go to hell, you goddamn bags!"

The two bathrooms in the residential area of the first floor are the center of considerable controversy among residents over when to treat them as public or private. Like the lounges, one is assumed to be for north wing residents and the other for south wing residents. This privacy problem arises because, like all other rooms for clientele use in the nursing home, the bathrooms have no locks. In addition, there is no way to notify others whether they are occupied. The dubious privacy of the "public" bathrooms has always made residents uneasy. However, this was never a "cause" at the Manor until one of its female residents, Joan Borden (alias the "newspaper," "Shirley Temple," the "general," the "sergeant"), who is quick-tempered and a prime gossip on the floor, was caught bathing by Don Staats, who is well known for his intolerance of and impatience with the "ladies." The incident, to residents, was the "last straw." News of it spread quickly.

Two residents describe the events that took place.

> But another thing I think is a mistake here. . . . There's a bathroom right here. Well, there's no sign or anything on that door. Well, how does anybody know? It isn't marked. So they know that there is no individual living there. Well, naturally, they're gonna push it open. They don't know. There's no sign at all. Well, there was a lady

—I think it was the "general"—was in there taking a bath and she stood up in the tub stark naked, and he [Don] walked right in. Well, now there's two sides to that. Maybe he knew that was a bathroom because he was here before I was. Now he could have done that purposely, and maybe not. But, I think most of them [male residents] are down there and I think the men should use that one down there. I really do. But it should be marked "men," and this one "ladies." There's no mark at all. So no one knows. I was here weeks before I knew that was a bathroom.

And Joan—you interviewed her yesterday up in the lounge—she was in there taking a bath and he [Don] was sitting up in the front there. And she told someone to watch. I guess the girl at the desk [nurses' station] was supposed to watch. She went down to the other end —the nurse—and all of a sudden there was screaming in there. And here she was, getting into the tub and he went in there to use that bathroom. She hollered to get out of there. I jumped up and I hollered, "You get out of there!" Here she is holding a little towel across the front of her, stark naked, and he says, "I don't have to! Who says I have to?" I says, "You better!" With that, the nurse came from way the other end and she, of course, talked to him and got him out like that.

After this occurred, a small social movement arose on the first floor. Several of the more outspoken residents talked with others about what should be done. It was finally decided that the social worker should be confronted with the incident at one of the regular meetings she conducts with the residents. At the next meeting, leaders of the complainants stated their case. Nothing was done about it. Several residents decided to boycott further meetings and informed the social worker that they would continue to do so until their desires were taken into consideration. This was effective in getting things moving. The social worker promised to have "bathroom occupied" signs made. She also took it upon herself to present a firm reminder to the parties to the bathroom incident that the Manor would not tolerate continued invasions of privacy.

The Third and Fourth Floors

The third and fourth floors at Murray Manor are generally more public to all clientele than is the first floor. Moreover, when a resident appears on patient premises, there are few raised eyebrows. The mood of public places on patient floors, such as the hallway, dining room, and lounges, differs considerably from their first-floor counterparts. The noise level is higher, and many kinds of noises can be heard clearly. A constant low din of moaning issues from some patients. At times, this is so persistent and monotonous that it becomes part of the taken-for-granted background of the floors. The staff that works fairly steadily on patient floors generally grows unaware of such noise, for, like sleep, it stealthily envelops a person until suddenly it isn't noticed.

Patient floors have more staff on them than does the resident floor. The first floor has one attendant at the nurse's station who acts and often dresses like a floor "hostess." Patient floors, being skilled nursing areas, are staffed by uniformed RNs, LPNs, and anywhere from four to eight aides. Staff work adds to the noise level of public areas. Noise includes bed-and-body work; commands to patients; staff exchanges along the length of the hallway; constant vacuuming, cleaning, disinfecting, and deodorizing by the housekeeping staff; and the din of patient call buzzers signaling staff.

Patients, unlike residents, tend to *fill* public places on their floors. This happens in two ways. First, for many patients, leaving their rooms and going "outside" means walking or wheeling down the hallway and sitting in the dining room or lounges. Many go "outside" throughout the day. Second, staff puts patients who have physicians' orders to be "up and about daily" but who are not ambulatory in various locations near the nurses' station, along the hallway, and in the lounges. There they remain, half the morning or half the afternoon, along with other patients and staff who interact with them or merely pass by.

Smells are no small part of the mood of public places on patient floors. There are four well-known ones: urine, stool, decay, and deodorants. Throughout the length of hallways there may be a succession of each, sometimes faint and sometimes pungent. These smells provide clues to the nature of staff work on upper floors at Murray Manor, namely, bed-and-body work.

As on the first floor, the publics of some places on patient floors are limited. Some patients consider it appropriate that patients use the lounge in the wing in which their rooms are located. Like residents, they invoke the lounges' alleged propriety in trying to dissuade certain patients from using the "wrong one." They use the same rationale to try to prevent staff from putting "certain sick and nutty ones with the rest of us."

The resident and patient floors differ sharply in the contrast between staff's and clientele's comparative definitions of the public limits of places on the floors. Some patients and most residents believe that the public areas on their respective floors have their appropriate personnel—not just "anyone or anything goes." However, staff's belief about this varies from floor to floor. On the first floor, it tends to coincide with that of residents. On patient floors, staff often treats public places as "wide open." This irritates some patients, who are apt to become rather angry about what they consider to be an affront to their sensibilities.

Several public places are not located on clientele floors. These too have limited publics. For the most part, lobby seating areas and the grounds are considered resident territory. At times, some places in these areas are even claimed as private resident territory. Except for a few patients whom residents consider "really one of us," when patients are present on these premises, residents tend to avoid them. They are considered to be frightening and depressing. Of course, residents rarely have to deal with them in these places since most patients remain on their floors.

The recreation area on the fifth floor is a public place. Many of its activities are planned for all clientele. However, residents —sometimes alone and sometimes in a group—are quite aggressive in pressuring the activity director to "keep the ones with no marbles" off the premises in their presence. Some residents threaten to boycott planned events if segregation is not maintained. A variety of sly remarks indicating their sentiments may be made to the director. Other residents, who are key links in the rumor mill that passes through most of the administration, are aware of the fact that the director knows they'll "bad mouth" the fifth floor if they don't get their way. Various parties to negotiations about the public nature of the activity area make it a percarious public place.

PRIVATE PLACES

Residents' Rooms

Residents consider their rooms to be off-limits to anyone but themselves and their roommates (if they have one). Anyone entering a room, be it staff or friendly resident, is expected to knock first and then listen for the occupant's bid to enter. This knock-and-enter routine on the first floor applies even to persons who are well acquainted. Residents take privacy for granted, for the most part. But notwithstanding the "code" of privacy, there are violations.

When Murray Manor was opened to occupancy, its very first clientele consisted of three women who came to reside in the north wing of the first floor. Because there were ample rooms available for future residents, these women were placed in semiprivate rooms without roommates, with the understanding that in time they would share them with someone else. As time passed, they came to command considerable prestige on the floor because, as they remind everyone, "We were the first ones in this place." Also, they are major links in the rumor mill mentioned above. Together, these women constitute the major clique on the floor.[5]

As rooms on the floor began to be filled, the social worker nonchalantly mentioned to the women that each of them would soon be getting a roommate. To them, this was the height of insult, since it threatened not only their private rooms but their prestige among residents associated with them. They mobilized to meet the challenge to their privacy.

The clique, as well as other residents, know that the home must increase its clientele census in order to remain solvent. The very first tactic in the battle for a "private" semiprivate room was to threaten to move out en masse. This would mean at least three and possibly more discharges, depending on who else could be convinced to leave. Top staff knew the clique had some influence on the floor. Members of the clique also contacted their relatives and told them that their peace of mind depended

[5] A fourth woman, Margaret Daley, arrived two weeks after the first three women and became the final member of the clique. Daley is the only clique member to formally contract for a private room.

on their having their own rooms. These relatives, in turn, begged the social worker and administrator to consider filling other rooms before those of the three women. Relatives' requests are usually taken seriously by the top staff, especially if the relatives are prestigious community figures. The tactics worked, and other semiprivate rooms continued to be filled first.

To most residents, Don Staats' behavior exemplifies disrespect for privacy. Staats has a kind of somber humor that the "ladies" in the residential area don't like. He also is not at all indulgent of the unofficial deference shown to the clique or of their territorial rules. Staats "pulls their legs," as he says, and they feel insulted. He has very low tolerance for "high-hatted, strutting" women.

As part of his usual rascality, Staats teases the women on the floor with his cane, pretending that he's going to catch their legs or necks with it. He also uses his cane to poke open doors along the hallway that are slightly ajar. This, of course, violates the tacitly agreed upon knock-and-enter routine. The ladies shriek, gossip, and complain for days whenever he assaults their room privacy in this way.

Residents who have roommates may have privacy problems within their rooms. This sometimes revolves around what belongs to whom. Although each room is clearly divided by a hanging curtain that may be either pulled forward or drawn, roommates do share a number of the room's features, such as the common sink, toilet, and window, which are permanent parts of the room, and the television, radio, and telephone, which are the personal property of one roommate but which may be used by the other.

Some residents consider that their privacy has been infringed upon when a roommate doesn't leave the toilet or sink in the condition that the other feels it should be kept. Some complain that they never feel that they have the private use of the toilet because a roommate's belongings are always there. One woman objected to her roommate leaving underclothing drying on the rim of the sink.

Through time and continued sharing, personal property that was once willingly shared with a roommate often leads to a privacy problem. Katy Miles, for instance, has a television set in her room that she invited her roommate, Joan Borden, to watch if she wished. Joan sometimes watches it when Katy is out of the room, changing the channel to one she prefers and adjusting the set at will. Joan's eyesight is good. Katy, on the other hand, has poor eyesight and has difficulty adjusting the set so that she can watch her own programs. When she is ready to watch the set after Joan has used it, she complains that "it's all fouled up." Katy feels that Joan is breaking her set and wishes that Joan would leave the set alone. However, she never shows her persistent irritation with Joan. Joan, moreover, continues to use the television, unaware of Katy's changed sentiments.

Roommate privacy problems among residents also stem from differences in daily routines. Someone who sleeps late may be annoyed by another who awakens at 5 A.M. Many residents retire as early as 7 or 8 o'clock. Some do not, and the early-retiring residents then complain about the "late night hours" of those who choose to remain awake until 10 or 11 P.M. A considerable amount of sleeping is done in nursing homes, and those few residents who do not spend as much time sleeping may infringe on the privacy of others.

Patients' Rooms

Patients have more severe privacy problems than do residents. Staff believes that the privacy needs of patients are not as great as those of residents since presumably, as a group they are less alert to the contingencies of privacy and, "after all, they don't seem to care as much about it as downstairs." When asked about privacy on the floors, aides on three and four typically mention that "most of those up here don't know when they're in their rooms and when they're out of them." Patients cited by aides as not caring about privacy are commonly those whom the staff considers to be senile.

Although aides generally believe patient floors to be more open than the resident floor, they acknowledge that certain patients do make demands on them for privacy. To floor staff, such patients are the ones that "have their marbles." As one aide mentioned, "They can make real trouble for you, if you're not careful."

Patients who are concerned about privacy carry a view of it that differs from that of the floor staff. Privacy-oriented patients are constantly vigilant over the boundaries between public and private places. Although they desire to maintain their privacy as residents, they cannot take it for granted as readily as residents do.

Both the extremely public everyday behavior of some other

patients and the generally "open places" attitude and actions of floor staff challenge privacy-oriented patients. Certainly, floor staff does take their sentiments into consideration, but staff's general floor orientation allows more violations of privacy—both by itself and by other patients—than it does on the first floor. When work on the floor is rushed, staff's "open places" orientation becomes less considerate of the privacy of privacy-oriented patients and of others. A heavy momentary work load means that the floor staff is busy dealing with specific jobs at hand, not generally scrutinizing the hall for patient decorum. Privacy violations tend to occur in such circumstances. They also occur when members of the floor staff are busy talking among themselves. Although this is not bed-and-body work, it keeps them occupied with things other than the affairs of patients.

Carrie Sopo is a third-floor patient whose room is near the nurses' station. Although she occupies a semiprivate room, she lives alone. The appearance of her room is extremely important to her. It must be, above all, orderly and clean. Everything is in its right place. Nothing is even slightly disheveled. Every morning, Carrie uses some of her fresh linen to wash her floor. She takes a towel, gets down on her hands and knees, and scrubs away. She always does a very thorough job—around and under the beds. There is a public telephone in the hallway next to Carrie's room. Occasionally, she scrubs it down too.

Carrie is one of the few patients on the third floor who keeps the door to her room shut. Her room is *her* private place. She works both to make it appear personally hers and to limit public access to it. When she is in it, she keeps her door closed. When she leaves it, she is very careful to shut the door after her.

On the same floor, two doors up the hall from Carrie's room, lives Sadie Saheen, a patient, who has difficulty locating her own room. From the hallway, all doorways look alike. From the doorway, unless patients have added highly distinctive accessories, they look alike as well. Although Sadie usually heads toward her own room, she often opens the door of, and sometimes sits down in, the wrong room. Carrie considers this error an invasion of her privacy, and it outrages her, making for periodic scuffles at the nurses' station.

The scene is usually the same. When Carrie leaves her room, she closes the door and walks down the hallway, turning her head and looking back at her doorway after every few steps to make sure that Sadie is not going into her room. Suddenly, Sadie comes out of the dining room and tries Carrie's door, ever so slightly. Carrie sees this from afar, rushes toward her, yelling that she should "come out of there." Sadie, always somewhat startled, loses her composure and usually shouts and swears back at Carrie. Immediately, Carrie walks to the nurses' station, looking back at Sadie to make sure she doesn't return to her room. Carrie scolds the nurse and aides there for not keeping closer watch of patients. An aide then explains to her: "We'll try not to let her go in. But, Carrie . . . Sadie doesn't mean any harm. She doesn't know what she's doing. She just forgets what room is hers." Carrie believes that this is simply an excuse. In anger, she answers,

> You should learn her to stop going into people's rooms instead of sitting around like little kids afraid to say anything to her. I don't like it and I don't think I should have to put up with it. I pay here just like everyone else. I don't care if she doesn't know. You should learn her! That's your job! I don't know what I'm going to do. If I could find another place to live, I'd move right away.

Castigating aides at the nurses' station is as far as Carrie's complaints about privacy go. However, Blanche Holden, another patient on the third floor, takes her complaints to the administrator and the administrative nurses. Blanche also is a link in the first-floor-dominated rumor mill. Her dislikes have a greater impact on the floor staff than do Carrie's.

Blanche, like Carrie, engages in constant battle for her privacy. Although she is blind and cannot see who enters her room, she has recruited several other patients along the hallway to "keep an eye on her room," as she says. They do so faithfully. Her systems works, for it catches privacy violators, both staff and patients. When Blanche is in another patient's room visiting, her recruits let her know if someone has entered her room and who that person is. If it is someone who has "business" there at that specific time of day, such as a housekeeping aide vacuuming in the morning, Blanche simply acknowledges the information. However, if the person has "no business" in her room at the moment, she quickly proceeds to investigate the situation.

Not only does Blanche strive to maintain her privacy by keeping her door closed and operating a system of room vigilance with the help of other patients,[6] she faithfully reminds the floor staff of its "duty" to keep people out of her room. These reminders are usually in the form of asides in conversations with staff in the hallway and at the nurses' station. As a symbol of her desires, Blanche has had a large sign posted on her door. It reads: "Keep this door closed." No other patient on the floor has one.

In general, on the third and fourth floors, patients who care about their private places must work hard to maintain them. The success of their efforts depends on their tactics. Some take advantage of such resources as gossip, patient support, and their knowledge of the location of administrators to get what they want. Although others have the same resources, they do not use them. Still others are not aware of these resources at all.

When patients don't work to maintain private places, they are not likely to have them any longer. This does not mean that they aren't desirous of them. Most do desire them, even those whom floor staff believes to be completely "out of reality," but privacy must be *made,* and on the third and fourth floors, far from everyone actively participates in the job.

The result of not working for or being unaware of resources to maintain private places is a relatively public everyday life. Aides gossip among one another and run in and out of the toilet where a patient is urinating. When one aide helps Claude Perlo to the toilet, for instance, he feels that he voids in private; however, when another aide stands behind her, he feels that the two constitute an audience. Laura Kowalski sits on a portable commode in the middle of her room, with the door open, obviously straining from the pain of a hard stool, with passers-by looking in. One aide laughs with another about "Sally shitting in Frank's bed while he watched," as they make the bed of an "obviously senile" woman who listens to their banter while sitting by her window. And Bertha Thomas' private telephone and television

---

[6] This has its droll moments. For example, when Blanche enters the south lounge, Cyrus McKain, her friend from across the hallway, often teases her by humorously reporting that he just saw "a couple of those women from the other end" sneak into her room. He then chuckles under his breath. Blanche, hearing this, scoffs and pokes Cyrus for making light of her. She then laughs at herself—half in jest but usually with the comment, "You have to keep your ears open around here or they'll take the shirt off your back."

are used by floor staff behind a closed door when Bertha is in the dining room or at OT.

In Public Territory

On the grounds and in the lobby of Murray Manor, there are no official private places, but residents do maintain "their chairs" at certain times of the day. Everyone knows, for example, that Cora Mommsen sits in the southwest chair in the side lobby during the early afternoon, reading her "stories." If someone else is seated there when she appears, another resident is likely to say to the one seated, "That's Cora's chair," or the occupant may say "Oops! Am I in your chair, Cora?" Such talk signifies a private place and sustains Cora's assumption that she can "act in private." Although no one need do it, and a few do not, most residents respect Cora's claim to that chair as hers at that time of day. In the morning or evening, Cora makes no such claim, although she may sit in one of the chairs in the side lobby. Even such trivial events as a temporary claim to the privacy of a lobby chair must be accomplished with work that involves mundane talk and gesture.

There are other claims to privacy on allegedly public territory. There are those residents who till "their" gardens; Joan Borden, for instance, tends "her" flowers. And the first-floor "ladies" have "their" time on the outdoor benches in the early afternoon. When the claims are accepted, these as well as other places are taken for granted. When they aren't, participants quickly become aware that they must work to maintain privacy.

CONCLUSION

In the following chapters, I shall describe the social worlds of varied participants in the Manor's everyday life—top staff, clientele, and floor staff. Each world provides its participants with a way of looking at and understanding daily life at the Manor. And each has its own logic: its own ideals, sense of justice and fair treatment, method of expedience, prescribed duties, rhetorical style, and proper mode of making decisions.

Place is related to such worlds in that it insulates one world from another. The designation of a certain location at a specific time as the private or public domain of certain participants tacitly assures the participants that a particular world of everyday life is being experienced there at that time. It allows the participants to take for granted the world at hand so that they can get on with business as usual. Places allow their varied participants to operate in seemingly contradictory worlds that look and sound quite reasonable from a position within each world.

The relation between place and social worlds, in practice, is more complex than place allowing for the rational conduct of a particular world. As I have indicated, some places are not well defined. This may lead their participants to assume quite different "logics" in dealing with each other, which, in turn, makes for what participants often call "troubles." What people say to each other on such troubled occasions shows evidence that they know of such entities as place and worlds, but only tacitly so. They may argue that "this is not the *place* for such and such." Or they may suggest to each other that as far as they're concerned (that is, their *world*), such and such should or should not be done. The remainder of this book portrays the complex relations between place and social worlds as participants of everyday life at the Manor experience them.

Top
Staff
and
Its
World

There is a way in which place makes absurd much of what is done in everyday life.[1] If you take persons who are, at the moment, members of one place, and listen to what they say and watch what they do, you will note that, for the most part, they routinely go about the taken-for-granted affairs of the place. It is meaningful to them in that it has some history of things usually done there. When its members happen to gather there, its meanings also are practical. "Being gathered" suggests to each of its members that, currently, there are things to be done and that a certain amount of seriousness is needed to accomplish them. Members may remind each other of this periodically when any one of them feels that the meaning of place is unduly changing. For example, they may remind each other of what the business at hand is and that they don't have all the time in the world to complete it.

[1] See Stanford M. Lyman and Marvin B. Scott, *A Sociology of the Absurd* (New York: Appleton-Century-Crofts, 1970); and Erving Goffman, *Relations in Public* (New York: Harper & Row, 1971).

If you take the same persons, but this time as members of another place, you will note that this place, too, has its meaning, memories, and tasks at hand. It also has its occasional asides, which invoke what is considered to be appropriate decorum. For its members, the affairs of this place, at this time, with such a gathering of members, seem as natural and reasonable as those in the preceding location.

Place makes things absurd in that what is done and said in one place is reasonable within it, but not necessarily within any other place. Members may talk about and do serious things in one place and then may "seriously" contradict the talk and deeds in another place. For example, they may seriously argue the diagnoses of particular patients in one place and in another place question the basis for even making them. Typically, they are aware of and take into consideration their seriousness within each place. But usually they don't systematically make *public* issue of the relevances, talk, and deeds of one place while in another. If they do, they risk the impatience and irritability of other members who, after all, "don't have all day to do what we're here for."

Like other participants in everyday life at Murray Manor, top staff carries on its routine business in certain places, each of which constitutes a location of serious, meaningful talk and deed. These places are top staff offices; administrative contacts with staff and clientele on the floors; and top staff meetings. What is said and done in one place at the Manor often strangely contrasts that of another.

IN TOP STAFF OFFICES

While at Murray Manor, I spent many hours in the offices of members of top staff, talking about a variety of subjects, including their work, which tended to fall into two broad categories: work that involved current and planned programs at the Manor, and work that focused more directly on clientele care. All members of top staff are concerned, to some extent, with both kinds of work, although some talked mostly about one or the other.

Plans, Goals, and Total Patient Care

In administrative offices, top staff refers frequently to "what we at Murray Manor are trying to do" and "how unique our overall program is." There are proud statements about how the home is coming to be held in high regard by various local and state agents. And there is persistent praise for the care program, its innovations, and future planning. But there is also very serious concern over whether desired goals are being achieved in the most efficient way possible. Top staff is eager to list its ideals and is not hesitant to state how it may easily fall short of them.

Top staff is certainly enthusiastic about its overall work performance. Its members have their personal disagreements, but all concur that the home is run by a "dedicated team." Although this is the administrator's language, everyone agrees with its sentiment. Somehow, in spite of the problems that occur between its members in their working relations, top staff believes that the ideal of having the "best nursing home in the country" run by a "completely dedicated team all running on the same track" can be achieved. All it takes is "good, solid effort."

The administrator, Mr. Filstead, compares Murray Manor with other nursing homes in this way:

> I've had the opportunity to travel around the United States and visited a number of these homes. I would say that what we have got here at this stage—we're probably far ahead of the majority of homes that are in existence. Any progressiveness . . . I think that the fact that we are not afraid to try something new, and it's never been tried. We know for a fact that in our drug distributions system, we're far ahead of the country. And, of course with our pastoral care program . . . just our requirements alone—requesting visiting clergymen to acknowledge their visits with the nursing staff and putting it on the charts is something that hospitals don't even do. I think the other key factor is that our medical director has a tremendous desire in the field of geriatrics. I mean that in itself has a great facet, because if he's that way, it rubs off on some of the people he's on the floor with.

The director of nursing also compared the Manor with other homes:

> I think it's up and above. I think we have more nursing hours than most nursing homes have. I think we have more professional people than a good majority of nursing homes have—LPNs and RNs. That's one thing that Mr. Filstead insisted that we do have. And this is one

thing that we do have is an administrator that really and truly is interested in patient care. Too many of 'em really aren't. They don't care what kind of care the patient gets as long as they get somebody in there to get money in.

Top staff members are well aware of what they consider to be differences between their goals and what they are doing at the Manor to reach them. They express faith in each other's abilities, but they also believe that, in many instances, their work leaves room for improvement. A few are dissatisfied with the patient care conferences. Some feel that various kinds of therapy services offered to patients are underdeveloped. Others believe that specific nursing cares could be improved.

In describing the conferences, the home's chaplain (who spends some of his time working in the social services department) voiced what top staff members believe to be a persistent problem in trying to formulate care plans for patients about whom they know very little. He said:

> Well, I question whether you can intelligently make a care plan unless you really know the patient very well. There's one thing that we don't have as much today as when I first came here and that was the seeming compulsion that we are now going to devise a care plan for this patient that will rehabilitate him. He will now overcome his difficulties. But, then, I sat there and thought, "Well, how are we going to do this with some of these people?" It wasn't a realistic thing. We are beginning to realize our limitations. If we do that and if we can face reality ourselves, and our ability, and how far we can go, I think we're making some progress.

The social worker also described program areas that she, and some other top staff members, feel need improvement. Like the entire top staff, she is optimistic about everyone's ability to improve.

> I'd like to get people doing what they're supposed to be doing, like get the priests in here to do their own thing. Or physical therapy . . . get these people into, you know, into patients. I can see where they're making progress, but there's so much that needs to be done. If

everybody just stepped up their own programs, I think we'd be a lot better off. It's a built-in kind of dedication on the part of the staff. They really want to make this place go. And this dedication really shows through. It's a very positive sort of thing. The patients realize it, the families realize it, and the visitors realize it. There's just a certain kind of . . . well, we give a damn. There's a kind of striving to reach some kind of goal, and facilities [nursing homes] where they don't have these dreams, I think that it gets stagnant.

The assistant director of nursing cited what she considers to be an area of nursing care in need of improvement.

The little things I come stumbling across, I guess, when I'm not there [on the floors]. I am not consistently there anymore. And very often it's later in the day. It's either very late or very early in the day when I do get any kind of rounds made. It used to be that, late in the day, I would find a majority of these things. Now, I'm finding dissatisfied patients, and disrumpled rooms, and, for instance, beds being made when patients should be cared for instead. Some of the girls on the day shift who at one time I thought were responsible nurses' aides are now not only undependable but I question just how responsible they are. The things we went through yesterday like occasionally hearing a patient spoken to in a manner we don't like—like things that need a lot of concern. Without that kind of concern, we don't have the kind of care we want.

It is clear from the comments about programs and planning at Murray Manor that top staff makes in its offices that it conceives of itself as fully in the business of building a fine nursing care facility. It has cautious hope for itself and for those who work in the Manor's varied departments. Its ambition is to improve departmental programs, not simply to run a nursing home.

Top staff's conception of clientele care has three important features. One is the definition of clients as individuals. Top staff has little or no serious concern with the social nature of life on the floors. Another feature is the idea of "total patient care." As top staff would say: "The philosophy and purpose of Murray

Manor is to provide quality care for the convalescent and aging person in an atmosphere conducive to meeting the optimum physical, emotional, social, and religious needs of the residents and patients." A third feature is the notion of a "sound mind," or, as they would say, what being "mentally alert" is.

When top staff talks about its work with patients and residents, it does so in highly individualistic terms. This is characteristic of its references to ideal clientele care as well as of its administrative practices in presiding over the care of patients and residents.

To top staff, good clientele care is care that is individually oriented. This means that the needs of the patient or resident are believed to come before institutional expedients. If a choice must be made between a care policy that would hinder the least able patient's well-being and having no policy at all, top staff considers it best to opt for no policy. "No client is worth sacrificing for the institution."

Whenever top staff talks about individual care, it typically contrasts this to what "many nursing homes" offer to clientele. As top staff members say, such homes are "just holding tanks for the dying" or "places where our senior citizens are herded with no consideration for their individual differences" or "big, impersonal places." Their ideals are clear: a nursing home should be a place that "does all it can for the patient"; it should strive to "be a warm, familylike place that really cares for its patients and residents." As the Manor's activity director puts it:

> The thing is, that you're gonna have to bend a little to what the patients need and want. I don't believe that you can write a hard and fast set of rules that would cover everything because you're dealing in humanity. Things have to be. Sometimes you have to play it by ear. You can't say, "Well now, the rules say this or that." I just don't think it can be done.

And its administrator:

> If we were doing something antagonistic that was crossing the winds of the particular patient, I think that it has to be dealt with on an individual basis. And I think the skill comes when you're going to have to talk to the physician, or whether it's a family situation, or whether

you have to outright confront the individual and be very hard and crack the whip with him or sit down in a very consoling manner or something like this. The trick would be . . . I think the real essence of professionalism is to know who you're working with. This is the key. And I think once you've totally missed the individualistic approach to the patient, I think you've had it. But that's a problem of our own.

And its social worker:

I don't think you can get answers, simply because everybody is unique. Every patient is unique.

When top staff seeks an explanation for a problematic client's behavior, it searches that person's individual background. If that doesn't suggest an answer, his "typical" personality is considered. Top staff overestimates the unity of personality to the detriment of considering social explanations of human behavior.[2] Top staff is faced with judging clientele behavior in three circumstances: when clientele are admitted to the Manor, in administering the care of various types of patients and residents, and in dealing with clientele "problems" that are reported by floor staff. In making sense of behavior, top staff typically is psychologistic. A few of its members, especially the social worker, wantonly use psychoanalytic language both to describe clientele behavior and to offer explanations for it.

When members of the Manor's top staff are asked the reasons for their decisions in placing newly admitted clients on one floor in the home rather than on another, they explain in the following ways. Asked why Hilda Samuels was placed on the fourth floor instead of the first floor, she is said to have a "background of paranoia." Asked why Hilda is diagnosed "paranoid" when she's never been psychologically assessed, the social worker reports, "From her intake [interview], it was obvious to me that she's the kind of paranoid personality that just couldn't cope with the freedom of the first floor." Asked why so many patients on the fourth floor are restrained, a top staff nurse explained, "Those are the kind of people that you just can't easily trust to stay put."

[2] Cf. Gustav Ichheiser's discussion of this in his essay "Misinterpretations of Personality" in *Appearances and Realities* (San Francisco: Jossey-Bass, 1970).

Asked why Connie Wodkowski's complaints about the behavior of her newly admitted, dying roommate are ignored, the social worker flippantly replies, "Oh, she's always been a complainer." Asked again about Connie's dissatisfaction over her roommate's behavior, the social worker says, "Connie's the type of person that you just can't really take that seriously, you know. Her neurotic anxiety about being here makes her such a self-centered introvert that it's hopeless."

Rarely does top staff seek social explanations for clientele behavior. It believes that people do things because of their personal desires or "quirks." Although top staff often *casually* recounts the interaction between persons that led to the particular actions of a patient or resident, such interaction is not given serious attention as an official explanation of behavior. The official causes of clientele behavior lie within the persons themselves, not in the contingencies of their everyday lives in or out of the Manor.

The idea that patient and resident behavior is basically a product of individual acts, past and present, influences top staff's administrative decisions about clientele care. The nursing care memos or care plans sent to the floors typically direct floor staff to deal with individuals, not with cliques, socially emergent situations, small social movements, or social ties. Directives may state: "Provide support," "Try to make more realistic," or "Get patient more involved in ADL [activities of daily living]." It is thought that somehow taking care of the individual patient or resident will reduce problems on the floors. When this doesn't work, top staff exasperatedly asks itself such questions as: "What's *wrong* with these people?" or "Can't they learn to adjust?" Persistent problems mean that there "naturally" is something wrong with some patient or resident on the floors.

Top staff does not seriously consider the staff and setting of the Manor to be integral components of clientele behavior. Clients make trouble *for* the staff and others, not *with* them. Clients should be helped to learn how to *adjust* to life in the home, not remake life in it.

Not only does top staff view clientele care in psychologistic terms, it also conceives of the care it provides as "total." Patients and residents should receive both proper medical care and attention to their so-called emotional needs. In practice, attending to emotional needs refers to whatever else besides medical care is involved in maintaining an elderly person at what is believed to be his optimum level of daily living. Officially, total patient care means providing for the physical, emotional, social, and spiritual needs of clientele.

Since top staff believes that total patient care presumably involves more than medical attention, it maintains that the Manor should not have a hospital atmosphere. As the activity director explains,

> You know, hospital patients come in and they're there a week, maybe ten days. But nursing home patients are entirely different because this is long-term. What you have to remember is that you're here day and night, month in and month out, and they get awfully tired of the same surroundings. That's why I'm having the birthday parties up here . . . and we don't give them a birthday cake or anything like that. But we do have a birthday party once a month. And we do sing "Happy Birthday" to each one who is at the party. If we have to sing "Happy Birthday" ten times, we do it, and mention their name so they know that this is their party.

Top staff wants the Manor's public places to look like home. This means various practical things. Floor personnel are asked to wear colored uniforms instead of white ones. Nurses are discouraged from wearing caps. Music is piped onto each floor to make for a "soothing, residential-style of living." Although it is not entirely clear what they are, activities of daily living [ADL] are encouraged. Patients are supposed to be dressed during their waking hours, rather than remaining in hospital gowns or sleeping apparel. Holidays are celebrated on each floor "so as to remind each and every one of them that they are still part of the world around them."

The administrator plans to make changes in some present arrangements at the Manor to create the "homelike atmosphere" that should be part of any total care program.

> I would put residential people in single rooms. I would not put two people together, for one thing. Well, I feel that when we put two together we've sort of discarded a little bit the homelike atmosphere and have maybe put institutionalization a little bit quicker in their minds. And I would not object if two people came in that had known each other for many years and wanted to live together.

I wouldn't object to that. But if I really had to do it, I would put them in a single room. So that would be one thing. The other thing would be that the dining room set-up would be much different. We could have family-style food service in preference to the present tray system. Family style will come as well as buffet and other unique meal services. But I would set those things up for one thing.

Top staff believes that the way to provide total patient care is to deal with what it calls the "emotional needs" of the Manor's clientele. Certainly, making the setting look "homelike" is considered important. But total patient care is believed to be more than this. As one staff member put it, "It's like the song says, 'A house is not a home until there's love in it.'"

When I asked members of top staff what they meant by taking care of the emotional needs of patients and residents, they invariably mentioned efforts they had made to provide a "home" for the Manor's clientele. I did not consider this a satisfactory answer, so I pressed further and asked, "Exactly what kinds of things do you *do* that fulfill these needs?" Their responses seemed to suggest that I was supposed to know what needs were and how they were fulfilled. They'd say: "Well, you know what I mean." "Emotional needs. You know, like caring for the person emotionally and spiritually. Letting him know you care." "Not just doing beds and taking patients to the toilet." "Stopping by to talk to patients and not just treating them like bumps on a log."

In attempting to describe what it means by total patient care, top staff makes frequent reference to the differences between working in a hospital and working in a nursing home. At Murray Manor, most members of the top staff had been employed at one time in hospital settings. All were negative about it. Some said that "you're just a pill pusher there"; others mentioned that "you're treated like a slave by the doctor." Many cited the "fact that you don't get close to the patients because you're too busy and they leave soon after they're admitted anyway." The implication is that long-term patient care in a nursing home allows the staff to become intimately acquainted with clientele. "It's more personally satisfying," one nurse concluded.

The administrative nurses and activity director noted a problem that nurses have in providing total patient care. Each reported that, until recently, nurses weren't trained to deal with anything but the medical care of patients. As the in-service director scoffed, "Oh, shit! If we got anything in the way of human relations training, it was just tacked on to the end of a course and forgotten." Top staff nurses felt cheated that they "were trained before all the recent concern for the emotional needs of patients." So, as one sighed, "You have to play it by ear and do the best you can on your own."

Top staff believes that it is seriously in the business of establishing "a solid base" of total patient care at the Manor. As evidence of its efforts, it cites holding patient care conferences (staffings), which strive to "locate the total care needs of patients and develop a care plan to put into effect on the floors"; periodically checking the floors to see whether the medical and emotional needs of patients and residents are being attended to; and "teaching the principles of total patient care to aides at in-service classes."

Top staff's involvement in total patient care is limited to administering it. Top staff feels that it is the job of floor staff to put total patient care into operation, on a daily basis, on each floor of the Manor.

Top staff formulates total patient care policy as if it has accurate knowledge of the individual medical *and* emotional needs of the Manor's clientele. Once formulated, policy must be made known to members of the floor staff, since they presumably apply it. Top staff believes that once policy is known to the floor staff, it becomes operational. Top staff periodically checks its effectiveness.

Top staff uses a simple language to talk about the problematic behavior of individual patients and residents. It consists of three adjectives that describe the soundness of clientele minds: "agitated," "disoriented," and "confused." Top staff *officially* attempts to avoid the use of "senile," which it believes to be vague, overused, and pejorative. As the chaplain says, "It labels people and I don't care for that."

This language is used to diagnose the individual behavior of patients and residents; this diagnosis then serves as the basis for "writing a patient care plan." By the way these terms are used, it is clear that they refer to individuals and are part of psychologistic explanations of their behavior. They are not meant to describe the personal effects of situational contingencies. In top staff offices, the meaning of these terms was considered to be obvious and clear. The director of nursing, Miss Timmons, readily defined them for me.

> GUBRIUM: What does it mean when you use these words: agitated, disoriented, confused?
>
> TIMMONS: [In reference to "agitated"] Well, usually we think about somebody that's wandering about, packing up things all the time and hoarding all the time, or incompetency.
>
> GUBRIUM: And what about disoriented?
>
> TIMMONS: Not in contact with reality. It can be time. It can be place.
>
> GUBRIUM: What kinds of things would a patient do to make you say he's disoriented?
>
> TIMMONS: Oh, possibly when you say disoriented, you think about living in the past.
>
> GUBRIUM: What about agitated? What would a patient look like who's agitated?
>
> TIMMONS: It's a wringing of the hands. Skin's clammy, usually a distressed appearance on their face.
>
> GUBRIUM: And what would a confused patient look like to you?
>
> TIMMONS: Bewildered. If they're truly confused, they're bewildered because they don't know where they're going, what they're going to do.
>
> GUBRIUM: Close to disoriented then?
>
> TIMMONS: Yes.

Mrs. Singer, the Manor's assistant director of nursing, also talked about the terms with no difficulty.

> GUBRIUM: What does a patient who's confused act like?
>
> SINGER: There's a wide variety here. It could be anything from a patient who becomes confused once a day to a patient who's confused all the time. And that's [the latter] usually based on a physical deterioration.
>
> GUBRIUM: And disoriented?

SINGER: To me, defining a person that way is someone
who is just not in touch with reality. They don't know
where they're at, or what the time of day is, or what's
happening aside from what's happening right this minute.
For instance, it's time to eat, but they don't realize it's
time to eat. You have to take them and sit them down and
tell them it's time to eat. Confusion means something a
little different to me. It means that they know that it's
time to eat in their mind, but they confuse issues and things
in their mind less specifically so that you know they're
not really interpreting things accurately, yet they're not
totally disoriented.

GUBRIUM: Do a lot of nurses and aides use those terms?

SINGER: Very regularly.

In its offices, top staff has "high hopes." Its members respect
each other's ambitions and plans for the Manor. Each feels, however, that there are problems that must be overcome before the
home can attain its ideals. Top staff believes that total patient
care is a fine approach to nursing needs, and that achieving it is
simply a matter of making a "good" care plan operational.

I shall now turn to other places in which top staff does its
work. The affairs of each place show evidence of being taken for
granted as reasonable by its participants. But when the participants' respective social worlds are compared, it is evident that
place plays no small part in keeping them reasonable.

ON THE FLOORS

In addition to its offices, top staff at the Manor fairly commonly
may be found in the basement classroom and in a small conference room in the east wing on the second floor. Top staff does not
often appear on clientele floors, and on the few occasions when
any of its members are found there, it is usually to complete some
administrative tasks, not to observe residents or patients in their
everyday life with other resident or patients and/or floor staff.

Top staff typically gives two reasons for not being able to
spend much time with patients and residents. One is that its work
as formulator of patient care policy and administrator of patient
care is "heavy enough that it keeps me in my office much of the
time" or "in all these damned meetings." The other reason is the

patient census. In order to maintain the Manor's solvency, the administrator continually pressures the social worker to "work on admissions." At the same time, he restricts the growth of his staff. As the rate of admissions increases, the administrative work of a stable top staff increases too.

The activity director complained about her busy schedule in this way:

> They really don't realize that I have to go to all three floors and get the people. And sometimes I wind up with a lot fewer people at an activity than there should be. And another one, Mr. Filstead, doesn't understand. He thinks I have all the time in the world. He really acts as if I have less to do than anybody else in this building and he has no idea. . . . Now like the charts. I have to keep track of all the hours that these people are in activity. This takes quite a bit of time. They keep adding more and more patients to the place. I have to get to them and talk to them. You can't be rushed. You can't really rush in there and snap off a lot of questions to these new people. You have to sit down and talk to them real easy and slow, and let them do the talking if they're able to. It all takes time. And very often they have a whole new interest, something that's not going on here. That's great! I'm all for it . . . starting something new. But, then, I have to try and match 'em up, if it's a [group] activity.

The occupational therapist added that the meetings kept her away from patients:

> Right now, I can't think of anything I'd change here. I'm involved in too many meetings. For myself, I'm not getting enough patient contact and I kinda really like that. It's just more of the organization, administrative role that I'm involved in . . . and that's because we're getting more patients.

The director of nursing described what, to her, was a typical workday at the Manor.

> Well, I usually get in here around six-thirty, quarter to seven, and if I can sneak in the door without anybody

catching me, I get up here and review the schedules and pick up the notes that are in my box down there. Who's absent? What's going on? What's happened? I try to review all the schedules before all the heavy traffic starts—the changing of shifts. If it's major, I try to get all the changes in the schedule and try to get other help for that. Then I usually go to the floors, and make a quick surface round. Sometimes I'll listen to a report and if I run into a problem patient or anything, I'll make some comment on it to the girls [floor staff]. And then, a lot of times, the night supervisor comes down and wants to talk. And then the day goes on. From there, I try to start working out the schedule for the next day . . . get that organized. I prefer to do that in the morning, then if I have to call the medical pool for people. . . . And then I check on the personnel. We have some evaluations to make . . . patient evaluations to consider like this. We have quite a few here that we haven't gotten to.

And then, it just seems like there's meetings all the time going on. We've had so many meetings. Sometimes I think this is one of our big handicaps, although he [administrator] has cut down on some of them. Every morning, we were tied up for two or three hours in meetings. Every Monday was patient care conference. Tuesday was staff meeting. Wednesday was policy and procedures. Thursday, we didn't have any because that was in-service. And every other Friday, we had something else. And a lot of preparation goes into those, whether you realize it or not—reviewing and checking it all out. Now, Mondays we don't have meetings at all, but Tuesday we have two of them. So, you practically utilize two-thirds of your day.

Then if you go to lunch, it's usually around 1 o'clock. Sometimes I don't even go out. Sometimes I stay right here. Sometimes I bring in lunch. Sometimes I go downstairs. Sometimes I sit in the conference room.

A typical afternoon is answering the phone, which can drive you up a wall. And interviewing people. Then, by 3 o'clock, you have changing shifts again. You have the same problems you had with changing shifts before. There's constant phone calls. "This one isn't in." "This

one hasn't arrived." "Are we going to have more help?"
Then, usually around four-thirty, things slow down a bit.
I don't get quite as many calls. So then I pick up things
and get things ready that I'm going to take home and do.
Then I usually leave around five-thirty or six-thirty.

Top staff is not delighted about being as busy as it is, although
this doesn't mean that it would prefer its work to be more leisurely. Far from it. This is an ambitious group of people. To
ask any one of them about patient care at the Manor is to receive a near diatribe of felt inabilities to attain desired ideals
because of "things we just have no control over." Top staff desires
to be less busy with administrative work because "we'd just like
to get closer to the patients." As the director of nursing ironically
commented, "Here I am. Trained to provide nursing care, and
pushing a pencil."

On most occasions (with the exception of death), when members of top staff are on the floors, they have little or nothing to
do with patients and residents as persons. They do greet them;
they smile; they may ask perfunctorily about their health—but all
this occurs "in passing."

"Passing" never takes serious account of others' wishes to talk
or gestures that signify a desire to exchange personal cares. It
can only afford the openings and closings of encounters. Those
who pass others are "busy" people with work that "simply must
be done." When it is on the floors, top staff deals with clients
"individually" by passing while it gets on with its administrative
work.

Passing, as a form of social interaction, has two sides. One is
brief opening-and-closing routines. In opening-and-closing routines, it is not usually considered sufficient that a greeting be
offered another person without provision for some, at least minimal, gesture of leave-taking. When opening-and-closing routines
are not fully completed, others are likely to treat those passing
as inconsiderate or arrogant.

Incomplete opening-and-closing routines have varied reper-
cussions for those persons dealing with others in passing. Those
who do not work to complete decorous routines may be sarcastically reminded by others that they have offered gestures of
recognition. For example, when openings or closings are not made
by a passing member of the top staff at the Manor, patients are

likely to complain to unspecified persons around them, "He's just too busy to say a simple 'hello'." Or they sometimes repeat greetings or good-byes to those who only look toward them in passing. I have also noticed that some patients may even chide a passer-by directly. For example, one resident patronizingly shouted after the social worker, "Now, Miss Erickson! We're not that rushed! Are we?" In short, among persons who are acquainted, encounters signify expectations of minimal mutual recognition.

The other side of dealing with others in passing is the business at hand. A decorous passing not only requires the completion of opening-and-closing routines, it also involves public signification that, in fact, there is pressing business to be completed at the moment. Public cues of this may take many forms. Loudly "talking business" while rushing is one. Waving various indicators of urgent business such as papers, charts, and the like is another. Pointing about intently at various physical features of place is still another. Such gestures signify to others that they can expect an opening-and-closing routine from those passing—and little else. It publicly legitimates very brief encounters.

When Mr. Filstead appears on the floors, he may be busy with any one of several things. He occasionally provides tours of the home for groups of outsiders. Sometimes he rapidly searches every wing of a floor for another member of the top staff who was reported to have been seen getting off the elevator on that floor. While on the floors, Filstead provides various clues to others that he has pressing business. He usually appears to be rushed. He walks rapidly; he looks briskly from one point on the premises to another; he often carries papers at which he glances as he hurries about. His face is serious, with a look of concentration and determination.

Patients or residents whom he encounters are dealt with in a highly stylized way. As he proceeds down a hall or as they walk by him, he offers exaggerated greetings to each one; "Hello-o, Mr. Canfield!" "Well, Margaret! Nice to see you today!" He often perfunctorily inquires about their health, and each inquiry is much the same as the next: "How are you, today?" "You're looking just fine, I see!" "How's that leg now?" He then signals closure with statements of approval or encouragement, depending on what those who have passed by have said: "Good! Good!" "That's just fine!" "Good to hear you're feeling better!" "Well, everyone has his ups-and-downs. I'm sure it'll improve." The intonation of these statements suggests that they are the *last* ones that will be offered. These statements are accompanied by various hand and face gestures that signify closure; for example, slowly but obviously turning his eyes or face elsewhere, or lifting a hand, palm outward, so as to suggest, "I'm done now. Halt and stay put as I go on."

The medical director, Dr. Cosgrove, also deals with people in passing as he goes about his rounds expeditiously. In his rounds, which are usually made monthly, he may be accompanied by one of the Manor's top staff nurses. The nurse participates in his opening-and-closing routines with patients who pass by him on the floors as he goes about his business.

On one occasion, Cosgrove is on the fourth floor seeing patients with his assistant, Dr. Samuel. They periodically return to the nurses' station together to make entries in the physician's section of patients' charts. At one point, Cosgrove is writing, his stethoscope around his neck, and Samuel and Miss Timmons, the director of nursing, look on.

A fourth-floor patient, Fern O'Brien, who earlier had obtained some milk of magnesia (MOM) from the charge nurse, approaches the nurses' station because, as she says, "It [MOM] won't work until tomorrow. I'm in pain and I want something for my bowels now." Noticing Cosgrove at the station, Fern asks, "Are you a doctor? Please give me a suppository. I'm so sore." Cosgrove briefly looks up at her, signals that he's busy writing, and returns to his charting with a look and gestures of finality. Fern is not satisfied that Cosgrove has heard her. Neither is Samuel, who informs Cosgrove that the patient wants a suppository. As Cosgrove increases the vigor of his charting, he tells Fern, "We'll give you a suppository if there's an order for it." Hearing this, Timmons looks at Fern's prescribed medications and whispers to Cosgrove that there's no order for a suppository. Fern, meanwhile, is listening to this.

After another minute of charting, Cosgrove tells Fern that there is no order for a suppository. She's heard this already, but Cosgrove finalizes the exchange by telling her himself. Fern asks him if he isn't a doctor. He says that he is but that her own physician, Dr. Thomas, has given no order for a suppository. Fern then concludes, "Well, I'd like an order because I'm feeling sore now." Cosgrove reminds her that she's had MOM and suggests that she drink plenty of fluids. He talks to her patronizingly and impatiently, without seriously listening. Cosgrove is determined to get on with his business, but he stills obligates himself to deal with Fern. He decorously looks down at the chart in front of him and begins to talk forcefully with Samuel about the patient being charted. Fern walks away.

There is still another way that top staff goes about its infrequent business on the floors and deals with patients and residents in passing. This involves opening-and-closing routines as well as talking *for* those persons who are being passed by. Staff does this when it feels that clientele will not be easily dismissed. One instance took place in an exchange between the Manor's social worker, Miss Erickson, and a patient, Sheldon Sykes.

Erickson is checking a few rooms on the fourth floor in the process of getting ready to admit two new patients. On her way down the hall, she runs into Sykes and immediately asks, "Why aren't you at the party on the fifth floor?" Sykes repeatedly insists, "I don't want to go to any silly party." Erickson, who is not prepared to spend time to entertain any of his objections seriously, begins to talk *for* Sykes as she pulls him toward the elevator: "Now, Mr. Sykes. You really want to go. You'll like it. You'll see. There'll be some nice cake and I know how you really want cake." Sykes repeats that he doesn't want any cake. It becomes obvious to him that she is done with their exchange when she leaves him on the elevator with, "O.K. I've got to run! You go up now and see what I mean."

KNOWING PATIENTS AND RESIDENTS

Top staff makes varied claims about its work. These range from claims pertaining to future planning for the Manor to those pertaining to the formulation of individualized, total patient care plans. Top staff's work related to patient care involves making care policy that is presumably based on accurate knowledge of clientele and their everyday lives in the home, although top staff has little or no ongoing, direct experience with clientele, except in passing.

Even though top staff is rarely on the floors, it does have some knowledge of clientele life, which it uses to do its work. The four sources of knowledge about the daily lives of patients and residents are their charts, information gained in passing while on the floors, anecdotes, and "serious interviews."

Clientele Charts

Charts contain two kinds of running accounts of patients' and residents' daily lives. One of these is medical. When a patient's or resident's physician visits him, the physician makes an entry, usually quite brief, in the physician's section of the patient's chart. Information here is mostly about current health status, medications prescribed, and possible new treatments. Occasionally, a physician may comment on what he or she commonly refers to as the "mood" of the patient. Comments on mood are typically stylized. For example, a patient may be described as "cheerful today," "appears depressed," "seems ready to accept his problems," "generally optimistic about himself," "unusually sullen," and the like. Except for the specific medical problems and treatments of each patient, physicians' remarks about behavior are fairly homogeneous, varying only in noting a particular mood.

Entering comments in their section of clientele charts is part of the physicians' job at hand, which is to check on their patients in the home at least once a month, the state requirement. Some physicians comply with this; others do not. As is customary after a patient has been seen, a physician records the nature of the visit. Physicians do not usually consider that their entry in the charts provides a systematic account of the daily behavior of a patient; rather, they record their momentary impression of patients' behavior along with medical notes. Once that is done, the physician goes on to his or her next patient. Like chart entries, physicians' visits to their patients at the Manor are brief and for the most part perfunctory.

The nurse's section of the chart contains another kind of running account of a resident's or patient's life. Top staff considers the notes to be a record of the important events of daily care on the floor. Aides are required to "chart" each patient assigned to them. This is done, officially, at least once at the end of every work shift.

The language used by floor staff in charting the daily behavior of patients is both personally and socially homogeneous. Regardless of highly variable floor behavior, the content of the notes is relatively uniform. I would have concluded after reading the notes that a single resident or patient, or at best a very few residents or patients, were being described.

In their notes, aides enter how well or poorly any of the following were performed: eating, defecating, urinating, sleeping, bathing, and walking. When any of these activities was performed admirably, it is noted in the charts; for example, "good appetite," "good BM," "slept through the night," and so on. When any was performed poorly, this is noted as well. If none of these activities was perceived as noticeably admirably or poorly performed, aides omit mention of them altogether and simply write, for instance, "usual routine," or "A.M. cares given."

The impression one gets from these entries on clientele charts is that, in the main, floor personnel consider care to be relevant only insofar as it refers to the care of the physical person. This contrasts with top staff's conception of total patient care. However, physical care is that aspect of its work that the floor staff perceives top staff to be "checking up on," especially in relation to itself. Thus, the information that floor staff provides to its superiors concentrates heavily on the bodily activities of clientele. Although top staff does not consider these to be its first priority in patient care, in *practice* it treats them as indicators of the quality of overall care.

The use of acronyms in any work routine is a clue to those aspects of work that most concern personnel. The acronyms most commonly found in the nurse's notes section of charts are W/C, BR, BM, D/R, SOB, and C/O. These stand for, respectively, wheelchair, bathroom, bowel movement, dining room, short of breath, and complains of. From the referents of these acronyms, it is clear that the bed-and-body aspects of patient care are critical ones for the floor staff. Even C/O, which could refer to a range of complaints from physical to residential and administrative, is most typically followed in the nurse's notes by descriptions of bed-and-body complaints and whatever may have been done for them.

The common usage of bed-and-body acronyms is not exclusively the product of how floor staff conceives of its accountability to top staff. Certainly, floor staff is trained (by in-service training, for one thing) in charting procedures. What is significant, however, is that floor personnel are also told, both by top staff and during in-service training that their job is the total care of the patient. Floor staff is informed that total patient care refers not only to the physical needs of clientele but to social and emotional ones as well. In spite of this, no acronyms with such referents are used. Chart entries typically do not describe social features of the daily routines of clientele even though they are often quite noticeable, and even though a good share of what floor staff deals with *on the floor* involves the social aspects of patients' and residents' everyday lives in the home.

Like physicians' notes, nurses' chart entries occasionally refer to the mood of a patient or resident. For example, he or she may be said to be in a good or bad mood, in good or bad spirits, or in good humor today. Where such descriptions appear in charts, their context shows fairly clearly that mood references indicate how easily floor staff proceeded through bed-and-body routines with specific patients or residents. If such routines were considered to have consumed an inordinate amount of floor staff's time due to what it refers to in the charts as "uncooperativeness" (sprinkled with "agitated," "confused," or "disoriented"), patients are described as having been in a bad mood on that particular shift. Such interpretation occurs on the charts despite the fact that when floor staff/patient interaction is systematically observed, there are a number of other obvious explanations for so-called bad moods. For example, some bad moods arise when aides interpret too loosely the bounds of mutual respect between themselves and clientele, thus *inducing* bad moods.

Aides' charting, which is left to the very end of work shifts, is usually rushed and perfunctory and is sometimes contrived. As aides gather about the nurses' station, all eager to leave for the day, patients and residents still call for service. Aides from the next shift tend to congregate at the station, too, although they do not consider themselves to be "at work" yet. There is considerable bantering between floor personnel. But in the midst of this, aides who are charting feel obligated to make an entry for each patient or resident.

When aides are rushed, they rely on the standard, reliable ways to "say something" about clientele in order to do their duty. Each always finds some way to say something about every patient in her charge that day. To all aides, this is just normal routine. As one aide described it, "You just do it. That's all. No big deal."

When chart information is compared with the manner in which it is used by top staff, things appear unusual indeed. "Serious" information about medical and emotional status and cares is gleaned from the normal, glib, routine paper work of physicians and floor personnel. Top staff uses chart information to formulate individualized care plans that "take into consideration the unique needs and desires of each patient." Chart information becomes part of psychologistic accounts of *each* patient's or resident's behavior and serves as the "factual" basis for writing *individualized* care plans.

Passing

Top staff also obtains information about the daily lives of patients and residents in passing while on the floors. Since top staff is much involved in ever-increasing administrative responsibilites, its evaluative function as work supervisors is a process of judging the quality of total patient care by quickly observing conditions on the floors. To top staff, good care is a matter of cleanliness and physical order (e.g., beds made, patients dressed, absence of odors). In practice, the most visible aspects of patient care are what matter to the top staff. Floor staff knows this and frequently mentions it directly in talking about its work. For example, aides caution each other about such things as "not spending too much time with patients when they're [top staff] around, but getting your work done." On one occasion, an aide who had been talking to a patient noticed me with a top staff nurse and said to the patient, "Well, I didn't really take much of a lunch hour, or my morning break, so we can sit down and talk a bit." This legitimized "sitting down on the job," since it presumably was being done on her own time.

When members of the top staff are on the floors, they sometimes comment on the quality of clientele care. Take the time Clara Johns died on the fourth floor.

As top staff is wont to do, it gathers at the death scene and presides over floor staff's death work. While there, Filstead takes the opportunity to "check out" the rest of the floor. After a quick walk down the hall, he returns to the nurses' station, where Timmons is standing. He says to her, "I passed someone standing nude in his room. I don't like that. Something should be done about it. The girls should be told about open doors." Timmons answers, "We tell 'em, but I guess that we'll have to tell them again. I'm going to have to have a training session with the aides." Everyone discounts the obvious. All other doors on the floor are open. It is common practice for all doors on patient floors to be open. As a matter of fact, both Filstead and Timmons take advantage of open doors in making occasional "quick rounds."

On another occasion, the social worker is in the process of receiving a patient who has just been admitted. She meets the patient at the front entrance. He is unable to walk and needs a wheelchair. Quickly, she takes the elevator to the third floor to look for one. When she finds none, she is outraged. For the rest of the day, she grumbles to other members of the top staff about the "poor quality of care upstairs." She repeats, "What's the matter with those people [floor staff]? Don't they have sense enough to know they need wheelchairs?" For the moment, she chooses to ignore the house procedure that assigns and charges wheelchairs to specific patients who are using them.

When top staff appears on the floors, it observes mere slices of patient/staff interaction. Rarely does it know or seek to know the daily floor history of an event it has witnessed. For one thing, it is not on the scene enough to observe the natural processes by which "unusual," "uncalled for," or "stupid" events emerge. Knowledge of such histories would make many of the events that top staff observes reasonable, but when top staff is on the floors, what it sees is interpreted and understood in terms of its own ideas and ideals of total patient care. If something observed doesn't coincide with this view, it may be considered a problem of floor staff's lack of concern for the needs of the patient; the quality of total patient care is at stake. The slices of the everyday routines of clientele lives and care that top staff does see are perceived not in their own right but through the eyes of policymakers.

Anecdotes

Top staff also uses anecdotal knowledge of patients and residents in formulating care policies and plans. This knowledge consists of curious and idiosyncratic accounts of specific persons and and of events in their lives. It is part of the daily talk of top staff members about their work "with" patients and residents and its trials and rewards.

Top staff calls on two sets of anecdotes to fill gaps in their knowledge of and explanations for clientele behavior. One set contains top staff's rich and vivid lore about patient and resident lives at the Manor. It is full of "dramatic" events that highlight and typify the behavior of certain patients. All top staff members know it well. When any one of them recounts these anecdotes, they are readily acknowledged by all.

Clientele lore is recounted in this way. At an appropriate moment, a member of top staff may begin by saying, "You remember the time that Fred . . ."; or one may start with, "Now, isn't that typical of Charlotte, like that time she. . . ." The other members acknowledge that they, indeed, remember by words or nods. As the account is concluded, they heartily laugh because the lore is often humorous. They may also shake their heads in stylized amused amazement that such things could have happened. "What will they do next?" "You never know with these people."

Clientele lore is absurd in that a brief sketch of an event in one context of an individual's life is used by top staff to typify that person's character in another context. Virtually nothing in the experiences that top staff has with patients and residents serves to contradict these typifications. And, what is more, with each recollection of an anecdote top staff is further assured that "we all know what [someone] is like." Its members actually talk themselves into delineating the reality of a client's character. Such "certain" knowledge, which enjoys full verification among the members, is treated as the "hard data" or "cold facts" of clientele behavior in top staff's deliberations over patient care.

A second set of anecdotes is not part of the common lore of top staff members but exists in the personal memory of members. Each one has a stock of "stories" about patients and residents with whom he has interacted at some time. These are recounted in a different way from the anecdotes that constitute clientele lore.

When the occasion calls for it, a member of top staff may recollect some event in the life of a certain patient or resident to fill a gap in knowledge about him. Such anecdotes may be presented by first saying, "I know why [someone] acts that way because I remember one time he. . . ." Or a member may add additional evidence that top staff is on the right track in its deliberations about a patient by interjecting, "Yes. That's true. Now, I recall the time she. . . ." Such recollections of personal anecdotes are received with interest, and all members appreciate the "light that your comments shed on this case."

As both clientele lore and personal anecdotes are supplied by various members of the top staff, a "rational" portrait of a client's character is constructed. The portrait that emerges serves to arouse memories about the subject "that I just forgot all about until now." Seldom does this portrait remind its users of "things" that might jar the reasonableness of the character being generated. What emerges from such deliberations are usually *"perfectly* confused persons" or *"completely* alert individuals" or "just *all-around* normal people" or *"totally* disoriented patients."

Interviews

On rare occasion, a member of the top staff conducts what is called a "serious interview" with a patient or resident. This usually occurs when someone has not met a patient or resident face to face nor heard much about him, yet is expected to take an active part in "filling others in" on him at a staffing. As the in-service director once said, "I just don't know anything about him and he's being staffed this afternoon." Patients or residents who are interviewed are likely to be either fairly recent admissions or, as one staff member guessed, "so quiet and to themselves that you'd never really know they've been around all that time." After the in-service director had completed her interview with a patient in preparation for a patient care conference, she concluded,

> I'm not too worried about the PCC when they call on me. I talked to Harry Fisher this morning and I know him. I'll go around and visit the rest of them [other patients to be staffed] so that I can get to know them too before the PCC.

The only thing that makes a serious interview different from a brief chat with a patient or resident is the interviewer's attitude. The client doesn't know he's being formally interviewed since top staff does not announce an interview as such. To the client, it seems more like a rare and usually welcome visit. Top staff considers interviews to be more serious than chats, mostly because it deliberately takes mental notes of what is said in order to use them at staffings.

Because serious interviews are publicly performed as visits, much of what transpires in them are social pleasantries. Introductions are exchanged; the weather is discussed; the Manor is lauded; the patient's or resident's appearance is praised; a coming holiday may be considered. In short, the interviewer obtains little or nothing about the patient's or resident's everyday life in the home. When the interviewer considers the visit pleasant, the patient or resident is judged to be "just fine." When the interviewer believes the visit to have been strained, or he is rebuffed by a patient, the patient is judged more negatively and considered to have a possible personality problem of some sort.

Interviews take place in various, momentarily convenient places. They may or may not be conducted privately. They seldom last more than five minutes.

IN TOP STAFF MEETINGS

Top staff formulates most patient care plans and policy in meetings. The one most directly concerned with this is the patient care conference (PCC). Once a week, top staff reviews the total patient care of two clients, each review culminating in what is called a "patient care plan." Reviews are usually referred to as "staffings." PCCs are scheduled for one hour, but frequently last longer.

The format of the PCC is simple. Prior to the conference, anyone on the top staff may request that a particular patient or resident be staffed that week. The staff member making the request may be expected to take major responsibility for summarizing that person's history. In the staffing, the patient's or resident's medical record is reviewed first, usually by one of the top staff nurses and in a fairly humdrum manner. Then the fun starts. Staffers begin discussing the behavior of the two individuals under review that day. Each member is expected to contribute to the discussion. This discussion consumes most of the hour, as those attending construct and reconstruct the etiology, diagnosis, and prognosis of the patient's or resident's "individual" personality. It is here that staffers utilize their "knowledge" of patients and residents with flair. Finally, each patient or client being staffed is summarized and goals for his care are written. Presumably, these plans are passed on to the floors and put into operation.

The following are excerpts from reviews of a few patients and residents. Regular staffing participants are:

> Mr. Filstead, administrator
> Dr. Cosgrove, medical director
> Miss Timmons, director of nursing
> Mrs. Singer, assistant director of nursing
> Mrs. Boucher, in-service director

Mrs. Smith, activity director
Miss Erickson, social worker
Rev. Edwards, chaplain
Mrs. Walsh, occupational therapist
Mrs. Hoffman, dietitian.

JOAN BORDEN,
SEVENTY-TWO-YEAR-OLD RESIDENT

SINGER: Joan's a very independent lady. She's quite active and participates in all the sing-alongs. The reason we decided to discuss Mrs. Borden is that she's recently had two strokes. She was watched closely. Dr. Savoy [Borden's personal physician; not present] feels comfortable at this point that she remain on the first floor.

Singer then reviews Borden's medical history, frequently glancing at Dr. Cosgrove.

FR. O'BRIEN [Borden's priest]: She's been very active at St. Barbara's. I saw her in bed here and then I saw her later when she was up and around.

TIMMONS: Mentally, also, she has deteriorated. She doesn't continue with her personal care. She has trouble with putting her clothes on.

Several participants nod in agreement.

SMITH: She has trouble with crafts. She can't see the calendar right. She seems confused.

A number of side conversations take place noting Borden's physical symptoms as evidence of her "mental deterioration."

COSGROVE: We should try to limit the demands on her. We should try to lighten an already taxed mind. This is not a time for new things for her.

SINGER: I'm worried about her activities outside the building. [Borden has planted and cares for a flower bed next to the building, among other things.]

COSGROVE: We should limit her outside activities. But I don't want you to take this as final. This recommendation is only for discussion.

SMITH: I find her considerably agitated. You know Joan.

TIMMONS: Her hearing must be getting worse. She
picks up certain things and interprets them wrong and
then spreads them. You remember . . . like she spread
the rumor that someone had died and spread that. [Alleged
death was reported incorrectly to the Manor's
receptionist. Borden overhead *correctly.*]

> *Chuckles. Many asides that recount various aspects
> of the rumor.*

ERICKSON: You're not thinking of moving her to the
third floor, are you?

COSGROVE: I think that that would be too sudden.

REV. EDWARDS: Well, I saw her helping someone in the
parking lot.

COSGROVE: Well, this indicates that she thinks of
herself as a leader.

ERICKSON: That's why we better be careful about
moving her, because we'd threaten her and she'd flip out.

FR. O'BRIEN: Joan, to my knowledge, has been very alert.

COSGROVE: I think if we should look at this over a
period of time . . . maybe we should lighten the burden.

ERICKSON: The family has noticed these trends also.
She's also a leader. When I first came here, Joan gave
me my first sock in the stomach. [Several staffers ask for
details.] She said that nursing homes are not for her.
[Other participants are reminded of similar comments
they have heard from Borden and recount them for the
staffing.] Now, she's a real promotor of Murray Manor.
[More reminding and recounting.]

TIMMONS: Miles [Borden's roommate] says that her
personal hygiene has gotten worse.

SMITH: I think she knows that she can't do the things
she used to do. She's had a few seizures. . . .

COSGROVE: By the way, we should get out of the habit
of calling these things "seizures." Maybe "spells." That's
bad too. Let's call them "thing.' Someone is having their
thing.

FILSTEAD: Father O'Brien, do you think these things
[PCCs] are helpful to you?

FR. O'BRIEN: Yes. I think that this is very helpful. We have a real practical problem in any church. When they go into a nursing home, we lose contact with our older members. So, when a funeral comes up, because of change in personnel in the parish, we don't know who this member of the parish was who was here ten years ago.

FILSTEAD: We do want you to be here at the meetings. You may agree or disagree with us, but at least you know what we're doing. You can get an insight into what we're trying to do here. We are trying to do what we profess to do when I first talked to you.

Considerable public relations talk. Borden's care plan is lost in it. Finally, the social worker interjects.

ERICKSON: [Rushed] Then the goal for Borden is to curb burdensome activities and encourage realistic independence. Right?

Everyone nods in the midst of side conversations about other affairs. Time is running out. The next case is introduced.

JEANNETTE BRUSKA,
SEVENTY-YEAR-OLD PATIENT

SINGER: [Reads medical symptoms from Bruska's chart.] She's a bit agitated. So the nurses think she needs more Valium. She gets depressed.

SEWELL [Third-floor charge nurse]:   She gets into what I call a "blue funk." She never smiles. She's always crying.

FILSTEAD: [Irritated] What's this "blue funk"? Is this a medical term.

COSGROVE: [Sarcastically] Oh, it's the latest vernacular.

SEWELL: She cries all afternoon until I get off work.

ERICKSON: What kind of approach do you use when you talk to her? Do you go in and tell her, "It's all right."?

SEWELL: [Irritated] No. I don't. Obviously, it's not all right.

ERICKSON: It just could be that the frustration is with her roommate.

COSGROVE: Let's have a physical/sensory evaluation first before we do anything.

ERICKSON: Maybe we should put her in some group with louder sounds because she's hard of hearing.

Considerable discussion among participants about how group work has "always worked" for them. Many examples recounted, some part of the Manor's lore and some personal anecdotes.

COSGROVE: But we don't know if she's hard of hearing.

TIMMONS: I'd like to mention a personal experience I had that's similar to Mrs. Bruska. Several years ago I had a carotid tumor and I was lying in bed. Some people came in and they thought I was asleep. They talked a great deal about my cancer and I was shocked because I didn't know I had cancer. I looked in the mirror later and I cried. But then I got mad.

Bruska's staffing momentarily is lost in varied inquires about Timmon's personal experience.

ERICKSON: Well, people, we're out of time. Mrs. Singer, you'll see that our goals for Jeannette Bruska [which haven't been discussed] are placed in her chart.

SINGER: Yes.

EILEEN RADKE,
EIGHTY-SIX-YEAR-OLD PATIENT

ERICKSON: First patient to consider is Eileen Radke. Dr. Resnik [Radke's personal physician] can't make it.

JANE SCHUMAN [floor nurse]: Trying to find things out from her is like pulling teeth. If she can develop a need to report symptoms to us, then we've something accomplished. She speaks of dying. She doesn't have a goal.

SINGER: I disagree with that. She has a very definite interest in maintaining herself at her present level. Jane, why don't you go on and give a patient profile.

Schuman continues briefly.

ERICKSON: She's an introvert. She's very family-oriented

and withdrawn. I don't want to put a psychological emphasis on it.

WALSH: She really wants to stay by herself. I think we really have to draw her out.

Other participants submit personal anecdotes about Radke that "confirm" her alleged introversion.

SMITH: She doesn't really feel depressed about being alone. It's a problem for us, but may not be a problem for her.

ERICKSON: That's right.

REV. EDWARDS: When I interviewed her this morning, I found no depression. She was really being very philosophical about her life.

This alters the character being constructed. Staffers now recount evidence for Radke's "philosophical" character.

TIMMONS: I see her as a very religious person. She takes a very existential role about "you die to live."

HOFFMAN: I've interacted with her at lunch. She's very concerned with the other patients' needs . . . whether they get their trays or not and so on.

ERICKSON: I don't think we should try to force our lifestyle upon her.

WALSH: Yes. I feel that if she wants to be alone, then that's her choice and we should respect it. Don't you?

COSGROVE: She may not think in terms of her body. The other possibility is that she understands very well what you're trying to do and is simply not clinically oriented.

ERICKSON: We have to think of her generation as different than ours. Her generation never learned to relax. Her life is empty because she has no work to fill it.

COSGROVE: Let's just treat her like she wants to be. That'll be our care goal.

FILSTEAD: What's the meaning of "treating like she wants to be"?

All staffers sigh and exasperatedly assure him that he knows very well what that means.

COSGROVE: I think that these conferences are good.

They enable us to get away from our bird's-eye view of things.

CLAUDE PERLO,
EIGHTY-FOUR-YEAR-OLD PATIENT

TIMMONS: Mr. Perlo's doctor has not seen him since his admission. His rehabilitation potential was limited. He's had episodes of confusion and agitation. For a short-term goal, try to keep him in touch with reality and to raise him to a higher level of behavior. Sometimes when I talk to him, he's improved, and at other times he's way down.

SCHUMAN: He had a really big conflict with his first roommate. Now, the present roommate doesn't offer him any stimulation. He'd go back to bed after ten minutes if he had his way.

SMITH: I've tried to get him to come to some of our activities. He says, "Get away from me with that foolishness!"

At this point, Rev. Edwards discusses what he knows about Perlo's railroad career. Then he and a few older staffers reminisce about trains and train rides.

COSGROVE: Maybe we should get another railroad man acquainted with him.

BOUCHER: That sounds like a good idea. That sure worked when we got those two teachers together. Remember that, Sandy?

Comments and joking about the "inseparable pair" are exchanged.

ERICKSON: Miss Timmons, will you read your long-range goals for him again?

TIMMONS: To bring him back to reality and participate in everyday life around him.

COSGROVE: I can see it now. Model railways and firemen's caps and gloves around. I'm serious.

Everyone laughs. All are talking about model trains and train rides

ERICKSON: Should we summarize Mr. Perlo and state

that we'll keep looking after him to see what he needs and how we can help him?

FILSTEAD: Maybe we can get him to paint model trains. You know—those little unpainted trains.

WALSH: I'm kinda against these playschool kinds of things.

Walsh's comment goes unheeded as others participate in the general light and jovial mood at hand.

SMITH: Maybe we should use model trains as a stimulus for all these railroad men here to begin to talk to each other.

ERICKSON: [Laughing] This meeting is degenerating.

COSGROVE: I think a railroad magazine sounds good.

GOLDIE KASKOWITZ,
SEVENTY-FIVE-YEAR-OLD PATIENT

SINGER: Cerebral arteriosclerosis. Possible CVA [cerebral vascular accident]. Babbles continuously. Enjoys being with other patients. Gives impression of being depressed. She should get some PT. She's on a Foley [catheter]. The doctor says that we should keep her up as much as possible. I think my goal would be to maintain her independence and keep her oriented to reality.

COSGROVE: Is she disoriented?

SINGER: The girls [floor staff] say that she's disoriented at most times but I don't know if it's the language barrier.

TIMMONS: She seems so lonely. I wish I could give her more time but I just don't have it. When I talk to her, she just lights up.

The staffing turns to other matters at this point.

WALSH: What I've noticed this morning at the reality session [A rehabilitation program to "bring persons back to reality"] is that Lulu Mills remembered Thelma's name.

FILSTEAD: We're going to give Sister Marilyn [the

Manor's receptionist] some extra jobs like passing out refreshments. Maybe we can get her to sit and talk with these patients who rarely get visitors. Do any of you have any objections to this? It wouldn't involve any therapy.[3] Just talking to some patients.

COSGROVE: I think that we should get our forthcoming spiritual director to coordinate this. Maybe Sister can get a spiritual history from the Catholic patients.

REV. EDWARDS: We could get more people than the clergy involved in the pastoral care program.

TIMMONS: You know, the Jewish people have more respect for someone in clerical clothing than even Catholics do. So I think Sister Marilyn really could help Goldie.

BOUCHER: What does she speak? Does she speak Polish?

FILSTEAD: Her son says that she reverts back to the old language occasionally.

COSGROVE: Then it's Polish.

FILSTEAD: We should have her son come in and discuss this with us. Her son is second in command in the County Welfare Department.

BOUCHER: She doesn't seem to be confused.

TIMMONS: She seems to be at times.

COSGROVE: Where is she from? Where did she live?

FILSTEAD: Knox Park.

COSGROVE: That's upper crust, socioeconomically.

ERICKSON: I'll contact her son and find out about her language.

FILSTEAD: I don't care about PR [public relations] generally, but I think we should take advantage of Alan [Kaskowitz's son] and let him know that we're concerned with his mother. Tell him that we'd like to know something about her language, and so on, so that we can help her.

---

[3] Top staff is quite sensitive about what patient/staff interaction is called "therapy" and what isn't. It considers itself to be the only personnel with knowledge of professional therapeutics.

WOODY SWANSON,
SEVENTY-NINE-YEAR-OLD PATIENT

ERICKSON: Will someone read the medical history of Mr. Swanson. Mrs. Singer or Mrs. Martin . . . I mean Sally Martin.

MARTIN [floor nurse]: [Reading from Swanson's chart] The patient's history states that he's confused at times. It says that he has full ambulation, but I don't think he should be allowed to walk because he's too unsteady. He fell this morning in the dining room. We should get a wheelchair for him. He doesn't want to be restrained and his family got very upset when they saw him restrained. [The chart states that] our goals are to improve ADL and treat his confusion.

SINGER: It's all right to not restrain him if the family will sign a form which releases us from responsibility should he have an accident.

ERICKSON: This man's social history is a bit more complicated than others here. He's well educated. He was a pharmacist. He's terribly frustrated and terribly embarrassed of being in a nursing home. He's going through a period of pseudo-denial. He'll get over this if we're firm with him and treat him fairly.

COSGROVE: Sandy [Erickson], what do you think are his ideas about retirement?

ERICKSON: I would think that he would have liked to continue his first-floor residency.

FILSTEAD: He was a Shriner. One of the reasons that he wanted to stay in this area is that his friends were in this area. Originally, his family wanted him to go to Green Lake in Bradensville.

TIMMONS: One of the reasons he clings to the first-floor ideal is that he had considerable prestige on the first floor. Some women were fighting for his attention, you'll remember.

All agree and smile.

SINGER: I'm afraid if we allow him to have that [wheel] chair, he'll fail further. This will go against his conception of himself.

FILSTEAD: I heard that some nurse on the third floor flatly said that he couldn't go to the first floor. That must have pulled his cork.

COSGROVE: Bill [Filstead], one of the things that's obvious from this discussion is that we don't know what this man is capable of. The purpose of the conference is to figure out, in a cohesive way, what the patient is like and what he is capable of. The basic problem is that we have a third floor. You know my position on this. I think we shouldn't have any segregation but only a small corner where our worst behavioral problems can be located.

GUBRIUM: How is his confusion manifested?

SINGER: I don't know directly. I've just been able to get this from the nurses' notes. I haven't had time to really talk to him myself.

COSGROVE: [Vehement and angry] This case has been very poorly prepared! I'd like to see it prepared further.

FILSTEAD: With all due respect, doctor, I don't agree. Isn't the purpose of these conferences to find out about matters we know little about?

SINGER: The problem is that I think that we're letting this man down. So often I've seen deterioration that's precipitated by anxiety that leads to confusion. I don't think we're giving him a chance.

COSGROVE: I think we should try to eliminate the use of these words, "confused" and so on. I do think that we should accept the physician's diagnosis that he's in physical deterioration. At least, that's settled.

ERICKSON: Reverend Edwards, don't you think that this person sounds like he's going through the denial phase of an adjustment situation?

REV. EDWARDS: Well, I wouldn't use these labels. But he might get a bit depressed because he's disappointed with himself.

FILSTEAD: I wouldn't mind if he came downstairs and had his meals with the residents. But you know what that would mean when we get more patients and open the other floors. It would just be utter confusion with patients and trays going every which way.

COSGROVE: Well, I do think that we should reconsider
this man. We do know that we can accept the fact that
his physician says that he's in deterioration.

SINGER: I really hate to see wheelchairs assigned to
particular patients because it just makes each person
dependent on the chair. Both the staff and the patient
begin to feel that it's easier just to use the wheelchair to
move the patient than to get them to ambulate. I'd
rather see a few wheelchairs on the floor that are used at
the nurse's discretion. Right now, all we have is one or
two wheelchairs of our own.

*Discussion drifts to staff problems at the Manor.
Nursing goals in Swanson's care plan remain as
originally stated.*

BERNARD OAKWOOD,
EIGHTY-THREE-YEAR-OLD PATIENT

*Dr. Cosgrove's assistant, Dr. Samuel, sits in on this
staffing. Participants are obviously aware of his
presence.*

FILSTEAD: We want to take the concept of nursing home
and convert it to health care. The modern home is now
a health care facility with modern architecture. We'd like
to get rid of the word "nursing home" and change it to
health care facility. We need geriatric care. There's just not
enough of it. It's here and it's going to be here—more so
than we realize. It's important to understand that in homes
like this what we're trying to do. We hope we can do it.
Hospitals have always thumbed their noses at nursing
homes. They're going to have to pay more attention to us
in the years to come. We are a good nursing home. But,
of course, we do have to face the problem that nursing
homes face because of the bad publicity. Well . . . I guess
I'm sermonizing.

ERICKSON: [To Dr. Samuel] In these conferences, we
try to discuss the problems, needs, and goals of the
patients.

SINGER: [Gives a profile of Oakwood.] Admission
orders are limited care. I've noticed considerable weight
variation from day to day.

RENSKA [floor nurse]:   [Whispered aside] That's funny.
I haven't noticed any.

REV. EDWARDS: I interviewed him earlier. I sat with
him at the breakfast table this morning and I found that
his speech was good. He seemed to be pleased that a
senior pastor visited him.

SINGER: I remember someplace hearing that he had
slurred speech.

ERICKSON: [Reviews Oakwood's preadmission family
situation.] His family was very upset with him.

TIMMONS: I think he has a sense of humor. [Recollects
an elevator trick that Oakwood played on her by pressing
various floor buttons.]

REV. EDWARDS: I don't know what can be done for
Bernie. [Suddenly becomes irritated.] I'm often asked by
the nurses' aides, "What goes on at those meetings?"
They're never told anything that goes on here and I don't
know what we're doing for these patients either.

    *Staffers become impatient with Edwards' brief tirade.
Sighs.*

FILSTEAD: Let's please get on with this case.

BOUCHER: [Aside] Does he [Edwards] think we have
all the time in the world or something?

ERICKSON: I think that Bernie is having a reverse
Oedipal thing with his son. [Oakwood, allegedly, is jealous
of his wife's affection for his son.] I think we should
prescribe diversional therapy for him and try to bring him
around to his real self and status in life. We have to work
on making him more realistic about the fact that he's a
patient and not on the staff. Mrs. Walsh, will you work on
that?

CARRIE SOPO,
EIGHTY-ONE-YEAR-OLD PATIENT

    *The following is an excerpt from a new form
developed by top staff to "format" the PCCs. Carrie
was introduced in the last chapter. She is the
meticulous guardian of her room privacy.*

Reason for Staffing: Inability of patient to tolerate any roommate.

DATA OBTAINED	SPECIFIC QUESTIONS
MEDICAL DATA: Gen. A. S. [arteriosclerosis], ceb. A. S. with transcient ischemic episodes; senility; ambulatory.	Past experiences and present attitude of patient seem to preclude double-room arrangement. Financial status would indicate need for this.
NURSING: Appetite good; sleeps well; up late; resists baths; cleans own room meticulously every day; very jealous of privacy.	Can relatives help her accept reality?
PASTORAL CARE: No contact with priest; declined any assistance in meeting clergy.	How long can we accept present unrealistic living arrangement of patient?
SOCIAL SERVICES: Believes son Tim (Los Angeles) owns the nursing home. (When challenged, she detailed his alleged statements carefully and without resentment.) Speaks of her second husband inconsistently (alive, then recently deceased.) Proud of seven children and how she sewed for them. Seems totally unconcerned about future	
DIETARY:	
OCCUPATIONAL THERAPY: Limited to few parties.	
PHYSICAL THERAPY: None.	

PERSONAL PROFESSIONAL EVALUATION:

Besides the PCCs, staff meetings are held at the Manor at which the administrative staff unwittingly makes patient care policy. These meetings are attended by the administrative heads of each department, whose official business, presumably, is not patient care; rather, it is "running the home." Issues discussed range from problems with the time clock to staff parties, the shortage of linen, the "mess" in the employees' lounge, and the cost of food.

Sentiments expressed in staff meetings may counter the Manor's professed claim to provide *individualized* attention to patients' and residents' physical and emotional needs. Some top staff members momentarily become aware of this and object to "regimenting the patients and our efforts to care for their personal needs." In most cases objections are dismissed, since "everyone knows" that the business at hand, in this place, is not patient care. As a matter of fact, those who persist (usually top staff nurses) in making public issue at the staff meetings of the affairs of patients and their care needs are ignored or cut short handily with such comments as: "Let's take that up at the proper time next week [meaning the PCC]." "This is really not the time and place to talk about these matters." "Let's have the nurses and the other disciplines take that up at the care conference."

Take the matter of air conditioning in the home. Each room has an air conditioner that its occupants may regulate and a window that may be opened and closed. This makes for cooling problems at times.

FILSTEAD: I know it's hotter than the dickens in there [Referring to the first-floor lobby].

MUNGER [maintenance]:   You're never going to cool this building when every stinkin' window is open. The curtains are open and everything.

SPARKS [housekeeping]:   Especially on the first floor.

MUNGER: [Disgusted] It's on every floor.

SPARKS: Isn't there a way of locking on the air conditioners?

MUNGER: Yes. That's the way it should be.

SINGER: But the problem is when there's a legitimate complaint of being too cool in a room, I can't turn it off.

FILSTEAD: When I first came here, I was pleased that we had individual air conditioners. Miss Erickson, maybe you can ask the residents in your group therapy sessions what they think about the air conditioning.

MUNGER: The problem is with the staff. Staff says it's too hot and residents say it's too cool.

FILSTEAD: Well, I don't think we should deal with all sides of this right now. We've got other business to take care of. Jim [Munger], see what you can do about it.

Another example of "regimenting" clientele at staff meetings involves the park benches located near the front entrance of the building. The administrator has been concerned that the benches, as he says, "bunch up" near the entrance.

> FILSTEAD: Mr. Munger, we have to be careful that the benches don't bunch up near the door. Maybe we should cement them down somehow.
>
> TIMMONS: Well . . . but they [patients and residents] want to sit in the shade.
>
> *Timmons is heard but ignored in the deliberations about the benches.*
>
> MUNGER: We'll get them placed down somehow.

I think it is important to note that what is believed by some to be regimentation is not considered by those accused of it to be so. Those "accused" sincerely feel that they are doing their best work properly. In response to their critics, they would say that you "just can't operate a good home that way." To them, running a home means operating "according to code" or "for the fire inspector's approval" or "by the rules of the game." Their good work in one place is insidious in another, though.

THE FATE OF POLICY-MAKING

When top staff has conducted what it considers to be an adequate appraisal of a patient or resident being staffed, it writes a care plan. Reflecting the staffing, care plans are psychologistic. They prescribe dealing with the patient or resident himself so as to alter his behavior in such a way as to make him, as staff would say, "more aware of reality." This means orienting him properly to the routines of daily life in the home as defined by top staff, and thereby reducing his alleged confusion. First, it is assumed that what is written will be carried out by the floor staff. Second, it is taken for granted that patients and residents will respond to treatment by changing their behavior along more "realistic lines." And third, it is believed that they will react to treatment as individuals and not involve other patients in receiving their own care.

The written care plan has two sections, reflecting top staff's concern with total patient care. One section, entitled "physical needs and approach," lists such medical directives as amount of ambulation permitted, feeding assistance, restraints needed, and occupational or physical therapy regimes.

The other section is entitled "behavioral problems and needs" and indicates the "approach" prescribed for them. Directives in this section are always sketchier than the medical ones. The approach usually prescribes treating the individual patient in a supportive manner to reduce his so-called confusion and/or disorientation; for example: "give moral support," "use a positive approach," "get patient to accept reality," "remind patient of time and day of week," and "encourage independence." In contrast to the relatively varied entries dealing with the medical needs of and approach to the patient or resident, there is little or no variation in the approach to emotional needs. The relative uniformity of entries for behavior reflects the way in which care plans are constructed. It virtually homogenizes clientele behavior and treatment.

The total care plan is placed in both the patient's or resident's chart and the cardex at the nurses' station. All floor personnel have ready access to these two sources, but they rarely read the behavioral problems and needs sections of care plans. They consider these entries superfluous to their work, since, in practice, top staff holds them accountable only for bed-and-body work. In the company of clientele, floor staff deals with events "as they come up" or "like anybody would." On the floors, there are no official "emotional" policies for each patient or resident.

Policy-making begins with the noble goals of individualized and total care. Top staff's lack of knowledge of clientele life and its psychologistic thinking homogenize the goal of individualized care. The nature of top staff's presence on the floors eliminates floor staff's concern for the behavioral content of the goal of total care. In short, while top staff busies itself with its affairs, life in varied places on the floors goes on.

CONCLUSION

Members of the top staff are the Manor's officials. Their view of the home portrays it, ideally, as a well-running system. When things go wrong, rarely is the system as an entity blamed. As they might put it, "A good home can be achieved when everyone pitches in and does his thing." When things are believed to be running under less than optimum conditions, people are at fault. The people must be changed from being too individualistic to being, ideally, parts of the organization.

The logic of the official view of the world is one thing; how it is expressed in practice from place to place is often quite another. As I have tried to show in this chapter, official practice among members of top staff may involve many characteristically unofficial acts and routines in some places that in other places are tacitly ignored in the presentation of the proper administration of total patient care. The logic of an official view of the home is used by top staff to present the Manor to themselves and to relevant publics in certain places. The same logic is unwittingly ignored, for the most part, in other places.

The Social Ties of Clientele

It is a peculiar aspect of social settings that their participants may see them in so many different ways. What may appear to one group as typical of a setting may seem trivial or undistinguished to another group. In settings in which some participants consider themselves officials and others clientele this becomes quite evident. Murray Manor is one such setting.

Recall top staff and its world. From its official point of view, all patients and residents seem to do what they do for the same reasons. Each is considered and treated as if the only thing he has on his mind is his own good or poor behavior. When it is mentioned that clientele have social ties both outside and inside the home, top staff members readily agree. "Obviously" they do have such ties, but to top staff this is so plain, it's not really worth making much of a fuss over. Officially, however, social ties are not part of top staff's concern with patients and residents.

Among clientele, much of daily life revolves around ties of various kinds. Ties influence the way they pass time, their personal troubles, and their knowledge of events at the Manor; ties complicate their lives. Indeed, a good portion of the "work" that residents and patients do at the Manor involves the effort to maintain or avoid social ties.

Patients and residents concern themselves with a variety of ties. When they first enter the home, the grief of breaking ties with home gnaws at them, and it continues to claim a place in their memories. Once they are established at the Manor, they guard their remaining home ties vigilantly. Occasionally, some residents and patients "step out" and reestablish their ties with the outside world. They go downtown, shopping, or just visiting. Among themselves, clientele have ties within and between places. On any floor, complicated networks of cliques, avoidances, friendships, and supports may be found. Supports are relationships whose ties are founded on the voluntary provision of help between clientele. Certain places on each floor, such as the dining room and lounges, impersonally tie clientele to each other. Patients and residents maintain ties with floor staff in varying degrees; some are friendships and some slight acquaintances. Clientele also have ties between floors, ranging from long-term friendships to kinship.

BREAKING UP A HOME

After taking up residence in the Manor, "all you have on your mind is what it was like back home and how you are ever going to make it here." With two worlds on their minds, one to which they are accustomed and for which they long, and the other an unfamiliar and seemingly final one, patients and residents commonly feel in limbo. The belief that a nursing home is a *final* place for one's life is what makes the idea of the place so frightening. Indeed, the belief is often right.

The smells and routines of nursing homes are, in some ways, much like hospitals. Clientele know this, for most have spent some time in a hospital prior to entering the Manor. But, as one patient said, "You can stand most things in a hospital since you know that it'll probably be over sooner or later." Their comments in comparing the two suggest that hope for a return to a familiar life and familiar faces and hope for one's self are what make hospitals tolerable places. Making peace with hopelessness is a difficult task, and it is the one people encounter in breaking up a home to take up life at the Manor.

What does breaking up a home mean? It may mean near total

loss of a familiar way of living. Although some describe it mostly in terms of losing others and their familiar possessions at home, it is their selves that are still clearly at stake. Take the following comments by clientele:

> I'm not adjusted to it yet. My problems were the loss of my husband, giving up my apartment, and getting rid of the furniture. It was a big job. I wasn't able to stand very good and get around the apartment. It was hard to decide what to give away and what to keep for yourself. There are quite a few "yes's" and "no's" you have to say.

> Now I get so mixed up ever since my husband died a year ago. He died before I had the [automobile] accident. My life is so mixed up that I don't know if I'm comin' or goin' once in a while. So I thought, "Well, I couldn't go home?" We live on the Lake—up on Smith's Lake. That's in East Columbus. That's about 30 miles from here. I'd never sell the place. I just locked the door and that was it. We go there on Sundays. I have no sisters, brothers, or anyone. I have nobody. I'm all alone. If it hadn't been for those two kids [her nephews], I don't know what I would have ever done. [Weeps] When Peter [nephew] takes me home, it's all right when I open that door and go in. But . . . when I lock that door, ah . . . [weeps] I tell ya, I like to go home, but not alone. It's a nice home. We built it when we were getting older. We had a nice home. I wish you could see it. We used to play cards in the den every night. And do you know there isn't any of our friends who live there anymore? Some passed away and some moved away. They have about six or seven children there now you know. They're so busy. That don't work. We have very nice neighbors who live there, but I'm still alone in that house. Life isn't what it used to be to me.

> And it wasn't easy after being, you know, living alone. It was hard breaking up a home that you've always had, you know, and entertained a lot. And I had a lot of friends. They always felt free to come in. Well, of course, it's limited here. I miss the activity [at home], but I

wouldn't be able to do . . . I'm eighty years old. I'm gonna be eighty-one and I know I wouldn't be able to do what I did before.

Oh, there isn't anything I don't like about it [Murray Manor], because I think it's quite a nice place. Oh, before I was living in my own home. Of course, that's the best. Well, your home is always the best. You have your own things. You feel better. Well, it's a matter of you have more friends, your relatives. You're not alone.

Well, I have no wife no more. So my son said, "That's about the best place [Murray Manor]." I was living with my daughter since my wife died last August. My son found this place. I didn't find it. He brought me over here. It's all right, but I ain't stuck on it. It's sittin' in the room all the time. Christ, you sit in here all day long. You go nuts. One of the ladies said, "You should get a little outside. You should take a walk down the block or two." I used to live over on Thirty-seventh Street. I could go over to the tavern there, and see everyone, and have a drink. I don't know of any places around here. But I just don't . . . I'd rather be by my children, or someplace close to them anyway.

Breaking up a home means losing ties with many people, objects, and places. Most recall the loss of loved ones—a spouse, children, a friend—with whom they once made a home. Their histories store memories of birthdays, weddings, and other times when someone, now gone, was somehow linked to them. Others reminisce and weep about the loss of familiar objects—a chair, a "lovely" dresser, a table—that they cherished and that were, for a long time, part of their lives. As clientele speak of objects, the things seem to come alive. Breaking ties with objects blurs a set of sentiments as does breaking ties with people. Leaving familiar places means that "all those things you usually do" in those places suddenly cease to be a routine part of life, and that all those familiar but unidentified faces of those places no longer form part of the background of everyday affairs.

Cutting ties with home is not just "losing the big things like your home," although certainly the loss of the "big things wrench a good part of yourself away." As some patients and residents sigh, "It's the little things that you really miss." The familiar trivia of everyday life are often the hallmarks of solid ties. The presence of trivial items, easily noticeable, assures one that, indeed, all is basically "as usual" in one's life. The long-term absence of familiar trivia is alarming, for it signals change. Two patients describe the meaning of "little things" as markers of life as usual:

> It isn't home here. I woulda' liked to have stayed with the children. We had a cat and I miss that cat quite a bit. I miss my little radio and the window I had where you could see the dog in the yard next door. Sometimes I really miss that nice little carpet I had next to my bed. I was used to that.
>
> _____
>
> I said, "Well, I'm afraid I can't eat that." I said, "If they had another biscuit or a slice of bread, I'd get rid of that little bit of jelly." But she [aide] never came back with that slice of bread. So what was I to do? I just put the little piece of jelly in with my straw. I like to drink milk like the kids do—with a straw. I'm not so hot on milk but I drink milk because I gotta gain my weight back. And I'll never gain it if I don't eat more solid food. So I took it. I got the jelly in the little jar in the top drawer. I thought tonight I'd take it down [to the dining room]. Maybe there'll be a slice of bread there or a biscuit or something. That's one of those little things I miss from home—kind of a tiny snack, you know.

Other patients and residents describe breaking up a home in contrast to their lives at the Manor. Rather than recalling ties with specific objects and events that have been lost, they see everyday life at the Manor as a situation without the ties of familiar places "back home." They refer to the institutional coldness of life in a nursing home. They cite the inconvenience of not being able "to do what you want when you want." They virtually pine for a tie with the "freedom I used to have before." As Toby Mann said:

> I don't think there's anybody that wants to be confined in his old age, but it's just a necessity. You all have to have a certain independence . . . to be your own boss, you might say . . . to do the things you wanna do and

can do. But when you're here, you lose that. You have
to learn the regulations, which aren't too strenuous.
They're fair and everything, but you have to eat at a
certain time. You have to get up at a certain time and you
have to eat certain food.

And Homer Wilson:

Well, this isn't home! This is an institution! You come
and you go. And well . . . it just isn't there. They're
wonderful to you and the surroundings are nice. They're
good to you, but it's still an institution. It isn't my home
regardless of how nice it is. They ring a bell when you
come in. They ring a bell and you sit down. [Sar-
castically] You haven't got a home. You have no place
to go. So you have to accept it.

And Martha Cush:

I just thought, "Well, it'll be a good place to live." From
the beginning, it was awful hard. Oh, it was very hard to
get used to it. It's just not home for me. But, I have to
put up with it and be here till I die. I hope soon. Very
hard. Very hard to lose your home. Just take yourself
being in my place. How would you feel? Think about
it. Just think yourself to be in a place like this. How
would you feel? It's very hard to take. Very hard. It
can almost heart break. 'Cause you got your own home.
You got everything in it. You do what you please. You
buy what you want . . . what you want to eat, what
you want to drink. Nobody in here . . . what they give
you, you gotta eat. If you don't eat, you go hungry. Lots
of times, I walk away hungry. It's clean. Sure. Everything
is nice. The people around are nice with me. Those that
do work, they do nice. And everything as far as that
goes is nothing to complain about that. But, as I say,
if I could help myself to be on my own, I wouldn't be
in here five minutes.

A final end to ties with what they believe to be normal living
is a hard thing to accept. It is felt to be very unjust. As one
patient asked, "Is this all I get for years of giving?" All feel

abandoned in one way or another. Some feel cheated by children; Laura Kowalski put it this way:

> I would like to go home if I could. God only knows if I will. I did feel terribly bad when they put me here, but . . . I tell ya, I didn't even know. I didn't. My daughter and my son and his wife and, you know, the relatives . . . when they were ready to bring me, all they did was get the Handicab. It brought me here and there was nobody here. They didn't tell me. There was nobody here. And I tell you, I did cry and cry. [Weeps] I'm sorry. There wasn't a soul here . . . not one of them. Nobody came along. Nobody. It did hurt me terribly much. [Weeps] I'm sorry. I can't help it that I'm crying.

Others curse the bodies that "let you down so soon":

> It looks gruesome. I wish I'd die. Then it would be over with. I don't see any chance of getting to the point where I can use my body. No, I don't make any plans. This damned body! I started feeling this way right after I had my stroke. No, there's no hope for rehabilitation.

Still others plead with "wretched life" for another deserved chance to return home:

> If we gotta be here, we gotta be here. But there is nothing better than home. If I could walk a little better, I would like to go home. Yes. I only wish for that, God willing. Oh, this awful life! I deserve better than this.

Underlying clientele talk about having had to break ties with home is an implicit sentiment of being shortchanged. This sentiment among clientele is based on their belief that hard work deserves its just reward. Clientele say this in many subtle ways. Some suggest it in the context of reviewing the accomplishment of having lived eight decades. They ask themselves, "And why should it end this way?" Others ask, "Have I been so bad as to deserve this?" They may ask God, as Laura Kowalski did: "God only knows . . . have I been so evil?" Or, while weeping, they may ask an unknown someone why their fate is such as it is, as Claude Perlo did:

Hello someone? Can you help me? I'm so lonesome. My
family don't come to see me. I don't know why I am here.
Why put me in here? I do nothing. I was good provider.
I buy good house and raise my children. I no rob. I
wasn't drunk or nothing. Why they put me here? I'm so
lonesome. [Weeps] I work hard. What happen?

MAINTAINING OUTSIDE TIES

Although breaking up a home means severing fairly continuous
face-to-face ties with a familiar world, it does not mean that
outside ties are cut completely. Patients and residents hear about
former aspects of their daily lives and occasionally see acquaintances in a variety of ways. Some are rather ordinary, such as
receiving visitors during the hours allocated. Others are rather
unusual, such as social ties that flow through floor personnel
who have contacts with outside acquaintances of clientele at
the Manor.

Some clientele have what seems to be an uncanny knowledge
of events in the lives of acquaintances "back home." It's uncanny in that it is so detailed and up to date without any readily
apparent means of communication.

When I first became acquainted with the Manor's clientele, I
looked for clues to ties with the outside. I asked about obvious
things: Do you have a telephone? Does your family visit you?
How often do you leave here to visit your friends? Answers came
easily: they told me how often they talked with or saw others,
and who these others were. As I became friends with patients
and residents, I was often present to corroborate their answers
when they saw others from outside the Manor.

Nonetheless, I was still puzzled by some of the knowledge
that patients and residents had about things "back home." On
every floor of the Manor were some who knew a great deal,
but as far as I could tell at the time, they had no way of getting
this information. When I asked them *how* they knew of the
various things that they related to me in detail, they would
typically report that they didn't "really remember [or know]
how I found out about it." At that point, I began to feel that
all this "news" consisted of tales-without-channels that patients
and residents "innocently" constructed, or that it was simply

an embellishment of old information. I concluded they had no ties with the outside world.

The "tale theory" of clientele talk about the outside world did not originate with me. It was mostly top staff's explanation of clientele news of the outside world without apparent ties with it. At this point, it certainly seemed plausible. After all, here we all were, in a place in which "everyone knows you have to take some of what all patients and residents tell you with a grain of salt."

As I became a more intimate and routine participant in the daily lives of the Manor's clientele, I began to discredit the tale theory of outside ties. This occurred mostly because my access to clientele life and my eagerness to understand set me apart from top staff. I began to realize that to know about some clientele ties, one has to be there when these ties are manifested, since some are so fleeting. Patients and residents, like people in general, do not keep rational track of all the mundane events in their lives. Initially, when I asked about some of these events I had assumed that they did. I also quickly became aware that a few patients and residents prefer to hide their outside ties; thus, when asked, they deny having them.

Whether their ties with the outside world are spoken of or relatively hidden, clientele cling to them. They are most eager to know "what's happening back home" or what's happened to so-and-so. On some days, ties with the outside world yield much information; on others, they do not. Regardless, the tie itself is cherished. I have seen patients crushed when an expected daily telephone call of less than a minute's duration does not come.

Ties with the outside world take precedence over any ties that clientele have in the Manor. Whether they are in therapy, at bridge, with friends, at dinner, or about to take a bath, they will typically take their leave or postpone a routine when the outside world beckons. This is expected. When a patient is known to have a visitor waiting, other participants urge him to leave an activity in which he is engaged. When it is known that a resident usually receives a phone call from her daughter at mid-morning, she may be reminded of this by others with whom she's chatting in a lounge.

Telephone links, routine as opposed to erratic visitors, and visiting outside are patients' and residents' most common ties with the outside. Patients' ties typically involve telephone calls and visitors; because residents are ambulatory, their ties are likely also to include visiting.

Telephones

To those who have private ones, telephones are considered "absolutely necessary." They serve as a kind of insurance that "no matter how you feel, you can always reach your people." Millie Ransom put it this way:

> Your friends call you and it's more homelike. I always had my own phone in my apartment. My friends call me and, once in a while, I call. My nephew's father-in-law had a heart attack and he was at the hospital. So I called them. He's back home now. I have an eye doctor and my regular doctor that comes in and different things like that, that I call.

And Martha Cush:

> I call some friends and some friends call me. Not every-day. That's the only one that I got. Who else could I talk to? It is important, if you got friends. That passes the time away. Otherwise, without a phone, you're lost. If you're used to having a phone home, then you come here. . . . When you had a phone home and you've been used to talking to people before and you come here and you haven't got it and you have no way of talking to those same people like you did before, then you're lost. That's why it's important to have it. If you ain't used to it, then it don't make any difference. But, otherwise, it's a right hand. Sure, a lot of them are sick. They can't come. So they call me on the telephone, or I call them.

And Bertha Thomas:

> Sure. It's important. That's the only contact I have with the outside world. I don't have anyone. Nobody comes. You're the first one that come in this morning. How do you like that! It's hell to get old. And I mean hell! Well, I know so many people and they don't come to see me. If that isn't hell, I don't know what is. If the good Lord

calls me and I'm put in the deep, it can't be worse than this.

Clientele are not limited to private telephones to maintain such ties with the outside world. There is a public telephone near the nurses' station on each floor of the Manor. Officially, clientele have ready access to them. Top staff assures relatives and friends of this "convenience which the home provides for its patients and residents." As the social worker boasted while she led a tour of the building for the relatives of a prospective patient,

> And here. [Points to public telephone.] The public phone is centrally located. If your mother ever has to get into contact with you for any reason, all she has to do is dial. And, of course, the nurses would be glad to assist her, if she needs it.

There are also two business phones at the nurses' station. Officially, these are for the use of nursing personnel on the floor in making calls to physicians, the pharmacy, staff on other floors, and the like.

The fact that the public telephones and those at the nurses' stations have officially defined purposes does not mean that in practice they are used in these ways. The social organization of making a call from these phones is more complicated than official procedure would warrant. Making a call may depend on clientele awareness that the outside world can be reached by means of the telephone, their having the money to use the telephone, their ability to complete a connection with someone they wish to call, and whether or not floor staff is needed in placing the call. In short, although use of the telephone is billed officially as available to any *individual* who desires it, it is actually contingent on a number of *social* factors.

Take the public telephone. When a client wishes to place an outside call, he first must know of the telephone's existence. However, not all patients and residents do, since clientele are not systematically told of its availability when they enter the home. Those who don't know of its existence but wish to make a call often "make trouble" for members of the floor staff, especially when they are quite busy with bed-and-body work.

Making trouble may happen this way. A patient in a wheel-chair tells an aide who passes him in the hallway that he wishes to make a phone call. To the aide and the rest of the floor staff, it's "obvious" where the telephone is. The aide tells him, "Use the phone," and quickly goes about her work. It's early in her shift and there's much to do before things quiet down a bit. The patient now knows there's a phone somewhere. He asks again, "Where's the telephone?" The aides nearby don't hear him, and he repeats his question several times, each louder than the last, with anger in his voice. Finally, although they've heard twice now, one of the aides in the hallway turns to him and ex-asperatedly dismisses him with, "It's down the hall! Go down the hall!"

The patient wheels himself down the hall, as directed by the aides. How far down? Where in the hall? He proceeds until he reaches the nurses' station, where there is usually someone to whom he can address a question. He tells the person standing behind the station that he wants to call his son. The public phone is pointed out: it's on the wall to the left of the station, across the hall. He notices it. Fine.

The patient, dollar bill in hand, asks the same person behind the nurses' station for change. She tells him that she has none but that he can get change from the receptionist on the first floor. He asks her if she can take him there. She doesn't answer him. She is buried in some charts behind the station. From his wheelchair, all he sees is the top of the station. He asks again, "Can you take me downstairs to get some change?" She tells him, "I can't take you. You'll have to wait till one of the nurses comes back." She is the unit secretary (ward clerk) and is not con-sidered to be on the nursing staff. The nurses and aides are on the floor distributing medications and doing "A.M. cares." He waits patiently.

A woman who looks as if she may be a nurse appears at the station. He approaches her. "Are you a nurse?" She nods. He tells her that he needs change to make a phone call. She says, "We're very busy now. Can you wait for a bit until I can get one of the aides to go for you?" He agrees and waits patiently.

His wheelchair is in front of the station in the middle of the hallway. An aide rushes off the elevator and bumps into him. She apologizes politely and says, "Let's move you over here out of the way. O.K.?" She moves him to the right wall opposite the station. He continues to wait patiently. Meanwhile, the nurse who asked him to wait has left. Other members of the floor staff gather at the station and talk together. He overhears them joking with each other and becomes angry. Twenty minutes have passed since the nurse who asked him to wait has left. She hasn't yet returned.

He wheels back to the station and begins shouting at the aides there that he needs change to make a phone call. They're annoyed. Although there's some debate among them about who is going to get the change, no one moves to take his dollar. The patient abruptly demands, "Will one of you go?" One of them takes the dollar and boards the elevator. She returns ten minutes later, hands him his change, and leaves.

The patient proceeds to the phone but is unable to reach the dial, which is on the wall three feet above him. He is rapidly becoming furious. As he wheels down the hall in search of someone to help him place his call, he sees one of the aides whom he had asked earlier about the location of the telephone. He yells at her, "Come and help me with this telephone." After a few moments of what the aide considers undeserved insults, she snaps at him, "Shut up, will you!" She pushes him roughly toward the phone, brusquely asks him for his money, dials, and nearly throws the receiver at him. He puts the receiver to his ear and listens. There is no one at home. He'll try later. About one hour has passed.

Aides avoid or deal brusquely with patients who they feel are unjustifiably rude to them. This patient's series of interactions with a variety of floor personnel has angered several of them. With each attempt to place a call, the hostility between them and him increases. He is rapidly becoming known as a "mean man."

Clientele must learn several lessons in order to maintain outside ties via the public telephone. The first is to know its "obvious" location; the second is to have the correct change. The latter is not easy, since having any money at all on one's person is discouraged by top staff. As top staff usually convincingly advises relatives when a client enters the Manor, "He won't really need any cash here. It's best to take it along with you rather than have it lost or stolen." Top staff has no desire to receive complaints from anyone, least of all relatives, about such matters as stolen money.[1] Should one need the help of the staff to get change or place a call, the third lesson to learn is to wait patiently for attention if one has not yet established himself as a staff favorite or has not become proficient in making good one's threats to report floor personnel to top staff.

Ties with the outside world maintained via the phones at the nurses' station are a slightly different matter. They are used by clientele under two conditions. In the first condition, since the station phones are considered by top staff to be for business only, floor staff is cautious in allowing clientele to use them. Two precautions are involved. Floor staff knows that top staff is most likely to appear on the floor from about 7 A.M. to about 5:30 P.M. Top staff does not work around the clock in shifts like floor personnel. Thus, the best time to break rules without being caught is after top staff hours, although clientele sometimes use station phones during regular top staff hours. A second precaution the floor staff takes in allowing clientele to use station phones is to have ready an account that absolves it from blame should the transgression be discovered.

When I asked aides if their superiors might object to allowing patients the personal use of station phones, those on the day shift typically would answer, "None of 'em are hardly ever around anyway." Those on P.M.'s would answer, "None of 'em are here. They're all gone for the day." I asked further, "What if they *should* happen to appear on the floor? Then what?" They'd answer, "Ya just tell 'em you didn't know she was using it" or "Say you're so busy that you didn't have time to run downstairs to get change" or "Just that she does all kinds of things she's not supposed to and that we've told her she's not supposed to use those phones." I have observed only two cases of top staff appearing on the floor while clientele were using station phones. In both instances, floor staff was absent from or turned away from the station. When one of its members was questioned about the practice, she accounted for it in a way I had been informed about earlier.

A second condition for clientele use of station phones is that

---

[1] Relatives may exert considerable pressure on the top staff since they are the ones who often decide whether the member of their family stays in or is removed from the home.

the patient or resident be a favorite of the floor staff. Floor staff is not as willing to "go out of the way" for someone whom it considers rude and offensive. Such clientele are told to "use the pay phone like everyone else."

Routine Visitors

Clientele also maintain ties with the outside world by having visitors. Visitors are more visible to other clientele and floor staff than are ties maintained by phone, and having *routine* visitors is highly visible. Anyone's routine visitors are likely to become part of the everyday life on the floors known to most participants.

There is a certain amount of prestige associated with having *routine* ties with the outside world as opposed to erratic ones. The prestige has two aspects. In relation to other clientele, a patient or resident who is known to have routine visitors gains prestige as a source of "social news." By this I mean that what routine visitors relate about events in the outside world with which the patient or resident was once familiar is not merely a body of information; it is also news that eventually becomes part of the daily talk by which clientele pass time with each other.

Take Eileen Schell, for instance. Every evening at about 7 P.M., her daughter visits her.[2] Clientele who are acquainted with Eileen, as well as the floor staff, know this routine well. The half-hour visit usually takes place in Eileen's room, although on occasion it's in the south lounge.

When it is about time for Eileen's daughter to appear, Eileen's friends bid her good-bye for the moment. Aides who pass her room often remind her that her "daughter should be here any time now." When the daughter appears, she greets other patients with whom she has become acquainted as she proceeds down the hall to her mother's room. Occasionally, she may stop briefly to inquire about someone's health or other such matters.

After her daughter has left, Eileen usually remains in, or walks down to, the south lounge for a chat with the ladies who gather there after visiting hours. Eileen reports in detail and with pride what her daughter "had to say." Much of the talk concerns aspects of this. Her friends ask various questions: "Is your granddaughter over her cold yet, Eileen?" "How's Peggy's new

[2] Visiting hours at the Manor are from 11 A.M. to 8 P.M.

job?" "Has Fred lost any more weight on that diet of his?" For a while, the chat is a fairly brisk one. Then it settles down to an exchange of judgments and commentary about Eileen's family's affairs.

On those rare occasions when Eileen's daughter can't make it for some reason or other, it is obvious to everyone. Aides ask Eileen, "Where's Peggy today, Eileen?" Eileen's friends are unusually quiet as they gather in the south lounge after visiting hours. When they talk, they "rehash" yesterday's news. They ponder various questions: "I wonder if your daughter had a better day at work today, Eileen?" "I guess she's preparing for that visit from her sister?" "I hope she's feeling better, don't you?" There is some speculation about the answers. The chat is notably shorter than usual, and they retire early that evening.

The other aspect of the prestige of having routine visitors relates to the floor staff. Having visitors who routinely come to the Manor visibly signifies that one has not been abandoned to the home. To clientele who have routine visitors, it means that they have recourse to some control over their lives, separate from the constraints of everyday life at the Manor. It provides some assurance that if all is not well in the home, they still have some reliable and trustworthy person to whom they can take their problems.

Ties maintained with the outside world through routine visitors are highly visible resources for clientele. They may be used at any time to influence the quality of their treatment in the home. Routine visitors come to know both people and various procedures in the home quite well, and what they don't like they are apt to complain about. The Manor's top and floor staff know this. It influences staff behavior when staff is in their company.

However, although clientele who have routine visitors know that such ties are resources, only a few patients and residents readily use them as such. For the most part, clientele *visit* with their routine visitors and floor staff manages to be pleasant in their presence.

Those few patients and residents who actively use their ties with routine visitors to influence floor staff's behavior regularly threaten to have their son or daughter complain to the administration about something that has annoyed them. Occasionally, they activate their threats. Members of the floor staff are wary of such clientele. As one of them said, "You just stay out of their way and you're all right." Floor staff is not as cavalier with such clientele as it is with others. "You just do what they want and get 'em off your back." As one aide explained, "When you're here a bit, you get to know who they are. You either run into them, or someone tells you about 'em. It's not that hard."

Stepping Out

A third kind of common tie that some patients and more residents maintain with the outside world is visiting outside. Clientele often refer to this as "stepping out." Stepping out is of two major kinds. One involves routinely visiting specific persons such as friends and relatives in their homes. The other involves such activities as going downtown once a week, shopping every day, or going out to eat once a week with one's old friends. Sometimes, one takes a bus on one's own to some destination; more often, a patient or resident is taken by car to a place he wishes to visit.

Like having routine visitors, stepping out has its prestige, part of which flows from the "social news" it provides clientele upon one's return. Like having a visitor, visiting leads to camaraderie when a person recounts to others the details of events that occurred while he or she was out. But another part of the prestige of stepping out differs from that of having visitors. This is the prestige of being *able* to go out.

Being able to step out signifies that there are persons that care to see one on the outside. It also means that one is not so poor as to be limited to the ties one has at the Manor. And it further signifies that one has the means to step out—a way to get where one is going and the physical capacity to make the trip. As one patient succinctly put it:

> The problem with a bunch of us here is that we have nowhere to go. And . . . if we *had* someplace to go, we couldn't get there anyhow. You really envy them who can go out somewhere once in a while. You know what I mean? You wish it was you.

Stepping out is a fairly ritualized and self-conscious routine. It is ritualized in the sense that getting ready to step out usually involves a fairly long period of leave-taking. Although residents and patients may spend equal amounts of time at leave-taking, what occurs and who is involved differs. It is self-conscious in that clientele are seriously concerned that they look "normal" in the outside world.

When clientele realize they are going to step out, they begin *taking leave* of their acquaintances and/or select members of the staff on their floors. This occurs in all but the most routine, daily cases of stepping out and regardless of how long one steps out for, whether only for an afternoon luncheon with the ladies or for a weekend visit with a son and his family.

The Announcement. The first stage in leave-taking is the announcement. For example, a resident has just talked to her son on the telephone, and he has invited her to spend Saturday at his home. It is now Tuesday. As she walks into the dining room for lunch, she announces the invitation to several of her friends. At table, they talk about its details. After lunch is over, she passes the nurses' station on her way back to her room. She pauses briefly to chat with a nurse sitting there. Before she leaves, she "inadvertently" tells her that she's to visit her son on Saturday. The nurse answers, "Isn't that nice of him." For the remainder of the day, she saturates all her acquaintances among clientele and staff with the news. Although she is excited, she makes the announcement casually.

Patients may make the announcement of leave-taking in a different manner. Those who are nonambulatory relate the news of their invitation mostly to members of the floor staff and to roommates. An aide may be the first to learn of it. From here, it usually spreads fast to other members of the floor staff, who are inquisitive about the details of clientele lives and gossip about them while on the floors and at the nurses' station. After the news spreads, aides and nurses are likely to comment on a patient's forthcoming outing as they drop into her room to complete one task or another. For example, as an LPN dispenses medication, she may say, "I heard you're stepping out tomorrow, Mrs. Morgan?" The patient nods and provides some details of the future event. A while later, another aide may ask about it as she stops by on her way down the hall.

The Rehash. The second stage in leave-taking is the rehash. Talk of stepping out does not stop once it is announced. Both the patient or resident involved and others continually remind each other of the forthcoming event. As the time approaches, staff may say: "I guess you're looking forward to Saturday,

Cynthia." "Now, Mrs. Morgan—don't get *too* excited." "I wish I was going on a fling." "Who's picking you up?" "Did you tell Miss Renska?" The patient or resident herself offers details of her plans for the outing. She may conjecture about what will happen and the varied dimensions of "how nice it will be."

The Preparation of Appearance. The third stage is the preparation of appearance. When clientele are about to step out, they work diligently to rid their appearance of as many clues as possible to their nursing home status. They prefer not be reminded in any way that the Manor lurks in their backgrounds. To them, stepping out is taken literally—out of one world and into another.

Various problems can make the preparation of a "normal" appearance somewhat of an ordeal. A patient who is bedridden most of the day may have to overcome a number of features of her typical Manor mien: no make-up, uncombed hair, sallow complexion, constant pain, incontinence, bed clothing, limited ambulation. When the event is considered a fairly special one, aides may work hard to help "normalize" the appearance of a patient for the outside world.

I witnessed several of these efforts, but the most memorable one for me as well as for many other people at the Manor, was the time Mary Clark, a twenty-seven-year-old terminal diabetic, was readied to step out for a Johnny Cash concert. Mary spends most of her time in bed, but occasionally she is wheeled into the dining room to eat or have a cigarette. She wears a urinary catheter, is very pale, and is in continuous pain. Her illness has nearly blinded her. Her "normalizing" happened this way. The concert is scheduled to begin at 8:30 P.M. It is to be held in an auditorium downtown, about three miles away, to which an ambulance will take her. She will be accompanied by two of the nurses from the fourth floor.

At midday, preparation to "normalize" Mary begins. Three members of the floor staff are involved at various stages: her hair is set; her clothes are neatly arranged; she is given a bed-bath; later, her hair is combed; two nurses apply make-up to her face; perfume is rubbed on her neck. The floor staff is very careful about its preparations. Finally, Mary looks like a youthful partygoer, except that she is in bed.

Mary is in a jovial mood. Her pain is secondary at the moment. She doesn't moan, nor does she grimace as she's moved about into her wheelchair. The situation she is about to enter is not appropriate for such gestures, and she manages to contain them. She jokes with Sally Martin (LPN) as Sally tries to pin a corsage on her dress. Sally says, "I'm so nervous, I can't pin it." Mary answers, "Why should you be nervous? You stick me with needles every day." An aide takes over and pins on the corsage.

The ambulance men come into the room to wheel Mary downstairs. Two nurses, also dressed in their "stepping out" apparel, follow. All three are excited, and except for the wheelchair, they look and act very much alike. In some ways, it's hard to tell who is staff and who is patient. At the moment it is time to be or to behave "normal."

As Mary is wheeled out of the Manor, several persons comment on her appearance: "Don't you look spiffy." "Wow! What a sharp-looking young lady." After the ambulance departs, more comments are made on Mary's appearance. One aide working on the first floor that evening says that she was "kinda shocked" to see Mary tonight: "Does she look different!" Later, on the fourth floor, another aide who had seen Mary depart asks an LPN behind the nurses' station: "What did ya think of Mary? You wouldn't recognize her, would ya? She's always so pale and moaning all the time. Oh well. . . ."

On another occasion, the business of preparing appearance to look "normal" while stepping out was the focus of a small social movement at the Manor. The movement, which lasted for about a week and was mostly a first-floor affair, centered on the wearing of wrist bands of the kind hospital patients usually wear.

When they enter the home, all patients and residents at the Manor are given such bands to wear on their wrists. The band is made of pliable plastic and remains attached permanently unless it is cut off with scissors. The band contains the patient's or resident's name and states that he is a patient at the Manor.

To many residents, wearing these bands is demeaning. After all, they consider themselves to be *residents* in the Manor, not patients, as in a hospital. They are very alert to the distinction. Most residents have grumbled about the wrist band requirement at one time or another.

Grumbling had been fairly quiet until two residents experienced what some referred to as "royal insults." One resident reported that when she had been out to dinner at a nice restaurant, "the waitress asked about it in front of my ladyfriends." And "I was so embarrassed, I could have died right there on the spot.

Well, I just decided right there and then that I had had enough. Off it came!"

The other resident, Homer Wilson, had been on his way downtown when he experienced what he considered an embarrassing situation.

I got on the bus and that's why I don't want that band on here. You're banded like a prisoner or something, you know. The motorman said, "What's that?" And I said, "Don't be disturbed. I just happen to be stopping at the present time at Murray Manor." I said, "Because my wife is there." I said, "This is just a little identification. If anything happens to me, they know who I am." I came home and took the scissor, and off! I'm not gonna wear it and I told her. I told Sister [receptionist] . . . I says, "I don't want you folks to think I'm getting pigheaded or smart by taking it off. I don't want it." It's a label that carries me downtown, and when I go around, they say, "Oh, what is that?" She said, "I don't blame you." Sister Marilyn said that. "If you wanted that on," I says, "to protect yourself, then you should have something that goes on the inside; something that's inside that is not seen." I says, "I would wear that." But, I'm not going to go around labeled like [Sarcastically]: "Oh, watch out for me! I might faint! Or, I might do something." Well, anyways, that's that. So, I will not wear it whether they like it or not. I'm paying here . . . and paying plenty. And this is my home and I'm a resident here as long as Mrs. Wilson is still here. While I'm going around, I'm not going around labeled. It's just your name and your address and that you're living at Murray Manor. That's all. Several people have noticed it when I went downtown or something. They'd say, "What's that for?" You're just labeled. You're going around labeled. "I am Homer Wilson—the elderly." They want to know who you are. "What you got that for?" "What's that on there for?" I don't know what they think . . . maybe that I'm an escaped convict or something. I don't know.

After news of these episodes spread to other residents, several of them decided to have a showdown with the social worker. The social worker conducts periodic meetings with residents on the first floor so that, as she says, "they can let off steam." Residents complained of the wrist band requirement at the next meeting. The social worker sympathized with them but persuaded most to keep them on for "their own protection." She also told them a number of atrocity stories of what might happen to them if they had an emergency and were not wearing an identifying wrist band.

The residents who weren't persuaded continued to grumble and argued that they would do something about the requirement. One talked to a top staff nurse to no avail. Another planned to see the administrator but, as she said later, "I just never could get a hold of him." Active effort to eliminate the wristband "requirement" for residents diminished after four days, although they continued to grumble about it.

The Farewell. The fourth and final stage in leave-taking is the farewell, which is usually more than a mere good-bye. Friends of the person stepping out are likely to caution her to take care of herself; they wish her a good time; they may compliment her on her fine appearance as she departs. Staff also may participate in farewells. They may tease humorously as patients and residents step out: "Knock 'em dead, Barry!" "Don't get too tipsy, ladies." "Look at the sheik! Watch out for those women." All who participate in bidding someone farewell imply by their comments that, for patients and residents, stepping out is not to be taken lightly and that it is indeed a somewhat extraordinary event.

Hidden Ties

Some clientele have ties with the outside world that are relatively hidden. These are more indirect than the ones discussed thus far and may involve members of the Manor's staff. Take Katy Lester, for example, a patient on the third floor. She has a telephone, which she uses frequently, mostly to talk to her sons and daughters, each at a certain time of the day. Her children usually call her. In this way, Katy, who is bedfast, maintains ties with people and places with which she is familiar.

Katy's brothers and sisters are dead, except for the so-called black sheep of the family. Presumably, no one hears from him or visits him. As Katy says, "My kids don't even remember what he looks like." She claims that the last time she saw him was thirty years ago. As I learned later, her brother had, as Katy reported, "very loose morals and got himself and other people in my family in trouble." Apparently, this led to a series of crises, whereupon a mutual boycott between the brother and the rest of the family emerged.

Katy talks incessantly about her family and daily reports details of her children's current lives to anyone entering her room. It was in this way that I came to know of her contacts with home. Occasionally, she interjects comments about her brother and what he's now doing, adding however that "Nobody has seen or talked to him for years." I ask how she knows what she does about her brother. She always answers that she doesn't remember how she found out.

After lunch one day, I happen to be doing rounds with Bertha, one of the aides on the third floor. Katy is assigned to her. We walk into Katy's room. She is reading the newspaper. After greetings are exchanged, Katy asks Bertha for the bedpan, which Bertha gets and perfunctorily places under Katy. This is all very routine. While Bertha tends to other things in the room, she chats with Katy. At one point, Bertha tells Katy, "I guess your brother had a little fall yesterday." Katy listens and probes for details as Bertha relates what happened. When the report on her brother is over, Katy says, "Well, I just guess that he deserves all that he gets."

I leave the room with Bertha, and as we walk down the hall, I ask her how she knows what happened to Katy Lester's brother yesterday. Bertha then tells me, "He stays over in that nursing home across the street. I see him at nights when I work over there. Katy . . . she don't like him. And he cool on her too. But they all listen. Yeah. They listen."

Bertha works the day shift at the Manor and P.M.s at the nursing home across from it. She learned about Katy's brother when Katy happened to mention his name one day in talking about her family. I ask Bertha why Katy always says she doesn't remember how she knows about her brother's daily life. Bertha tells me that Katy always says that because she doesn't want anyone to know she has any contact with him.

Some ties with the outside world are maintained through other patients' and residents' visitors. Some patients and residents at the Manor are hardly ever visited by friends or relatives from outside the home. They don't have telephones. Their lives at the

Manor are, for the most part, fairly isolated as far as the outside world is concerned.

Anna Vukovich is one of the Manor's isolated patients. Her daily life on the fourth floor is limited to what staff calls activities of daily living (ADL). She practices these (eating, sleeping, resting, chatting, voiding) in the nursing home every day, year round. Anna's conversations are time-erratic. At one moment, she may be chatting about her childhood; at another, she talks in detail about what her husband and sons are now doing. As she goes from one topic to another, she does not provide her listener with any obvious transition cues. This has further isolated her at the Manor since, as both staff and patients would say, "You can't talk with her. What's the use? She gets everything mixed up." Furthermore, all believe that when she talks about her family, "you know it's all nonsense or she makes it up." As an aide commented, "How could she know? Her family has abandoned her. I know for a fact that no one visits her. She's just all turned around."

Two doors down from Anna's room is a patient who enjoys daily visits from her daughters. As is common, the daughters have made the acquaintance of other patients on the floor as well as of the visitors of other patients. They know Anna. But what is significant for outside ties is that they also know Anna's family. Both families are members of the same parish and reside in the same neighborhood.

When the daughters visit their mother, they also politely greet and briefly chat with other patients on the floor with whom they are acquainted. When Anna encounters the daughters, she is delighted. She eagerly asks about her sons and husband—what they are doing now, what they did yesterday, and what their plans are for tomorrow. The daughters sympathetically oblige. She always asks the daughters whether they think her sons will visit her, and they always politely answer that they "probably will visit any day now." The sons never do. This encounter takes place almost daily. It is short, usually lasting for only a few minutes. It is the way that Anna maintains ties with home. What she later relates to other patients and staff about her family's current affairs are detailed and fairly accurate recollections of the daughters' reports. However, everyone knows that Anna never sees or talks to her family.

Anna's way of maintaining outside ties is not unusual at the Manor. It is in part an accidental outcome of the way in which nursing homes are chosen. In a sense, this is like ethnic migration. When a family has selected the Manor as a place for its elder, it oftens informs other families with elders. Or a priest who has one former parishioner at the Manor may encourage other parishioners to place their elders there.

Patients and residents may keep outside ties through the outside visiting of other clientele. In some instances, this kind of tie is highly routinized. Upon the return of a patient or resident who has visited home, a relatively isolated acquaintance of his may ask, "What's new?" What may ensue are short reports about the current status of people and places with which both were acquainted before coming to live at the Manor. The following brief exchange typifies such reports.

PATIENT A: Hi, George.

PATIENT B: How's everything on the old home front?

PATIENT A: Not bad. I passed by your place. It looks the same as when you was home.

PATIENT B: I guess they're taking care of it. They're not a bad bunch of kids. Eh, Mike?

PATIENT A: You can say that again. A new family moved in down your street. They look Mexican or something.

PATIENT B: Yeah?

MAINTAINING INSIDE TIES

The world of patients and residents inside the Manor involves a network of social ties and avoidances. Much of their talk and deeds are part and parcel of this network. Although this network extends from one floor to another, it is within the confines of each floor that it is most complex.

Cliques

On each floor of the Manor there are cliques—groups of clientele whose members consider themselves special in some way. The clique serves to identify its members as separate from other patients or residents. In their talk, the members make a point of two differences. First, members of a clique talk concertedly about what identifies them as a group separate from others. Second, they also talk about those outside the clique and what identifies them as not qualified for membership. Being identified as a special group, members behave in a special way. They work to maintain their solidarity. On the floors of the Manor, this is very much an affair of place.

Although both patients and residents maintain cliques, their bases of solidarity differ. Patients who are members of cliques consider themselves special because they believe they are more alert than other patients. Residents do not integrate themselves into cliques for this reason. Alertness is not a criterion for clique membership among residents. After all, as they would say, "The first floor is for those who have their marbles." Rather, residents who belong to cliques claim special distinction because, for example, they have been at the Manor longer than anyone else, or they smoke, or they play certain card games well.

Patient Cliques. Members of the patient alertness cliques often reside in proximate areas of the hallway. One of the most obvious clues to their existence are references to the relative mental competence of members as opposed to other patients. Members' conversations are filled with such references. Those in alertness cliques refer to themselves as the sane ones, we who have our marbles, alert, those who have minds. knowing what's going on, and having it right up in the head. They refer to other patients as nutty, hoopty doopty, those you feel sorry for, the poor things, loonies, senile, those without their marbles, not all there, mindless, and goofy. The following excerpts from clique members' conversations exemplify these distinctions:

> I avoid all of them because you can't communicate with them. You say something in a sentence and the nuts will look at you and say "slkjlrhtlsrlsk!#%°" And I ask 'em what they're saying and they say it over again. I don't know what they're saying. So, what's the use. The ones I've talked to are like that.
>
> ———
>
> I didn't realize the conditions of the minds on this floor. There's only a few that you can talk to. It makes me feel as though I've been railroaded into an asylum. That hurts me mentally, you know. I can't, uh. . . . If I felt well, I would be the most sympathetic person in the world and help every chance I get.
>
> ———
>
> I think they're all good people. But, I feel so sorry for

some of them. I think some of 'em start feeling upset when it gets near nightfall. I don't know why, but they do.

_____

Well, I don't go here and talk to any of them with half their heads chopped off. You know what I mean. They can't think and they can't do. Some of us are too bright for that. They don't bother me. I don't talk to them. I leave 'em alone.

_____

About living together with roommates . . . normal people should be separate and senile people too because they understand each other. And we understand each other too. So we can live better that way. Before I used to go out to the sun room [south lounge] and sit there. Lately, I didn't go there. Just for two weeks, I didn't go there at all. Well, because there are too many senile . . . no marbles. . . . The nurses bring them in there and they holler and cry. "Help me, please! Help me! Help me!" And the nurses don't help them. So we ladies [members of the alertness clique] have to go to whatever was the closest room till the nurses came over and take them out. I think those that are senile and very sick should be separate and those that are healthy and with good minds should be kept separate too.

The most well-developed way of distinguishing between members and nonmembers are "marble" references. They lend themselves to finer distinctions than references to whether or not a person is senile. Patients outside of cliques who are considered to be the most mentally incompetent are said to have lost all their marbles. Those judged to have some ability to communicate are said to have a few of their marbles left. Any clique patient who, for one reason or another, "makes trouble" for any other is said to be losing his marbles. Finally, members in good standing of the alertness cliques are believed to have all their marbles.[3]

Among patients, the business of whether or not one is consid-

_____

[3] Floor staff and residents also use references to "marbles" but not usually to delineate members and nonmembers of alertness cliques. Floor staff uses such references to distinguish the kind of patient it has to treat delicately from other kinds. Residents use references to "marbles" to make distinctions between floors.

ered to have his marbles affects who associates with whom. Clique ties are guarded vigilantly on the floor. Wherever they are manifested, that place is considered out of bounds for nonmembers.

Although officially the north and south lounges at the Manor are for any patient's use, on the floors there is a working understanding that patients use the one nearest to their room. Both patients and floor staff tend to adhere to this. First of all, it coincides with many patients' inability to walk "all the way to the other end without getting tired." Second, it supports floor staff's attempt to keep the floor in order, which to some extent means patients "staying put" or "knowing their whereabouts."

In addition, members of alertness cliques believe that their presence in the lounges should be honored by the floor staff. Although members don't claim the lounges as their exclusive territory, they do believe that when they are present there, so-called senile patients should be elsewhere. Likewise, when senile patients are using a lounge, members avoid using it. As they would say, "It's only fair to everyone that they should be separate."

Floor staff does not strictly honor clique separation sentiments. Its main concern is getting through bed-and-body work, which it judges to be progressing well when patients "stay put" and do not unduly disrupt what it considers normal floor routine. What floor staff considers "staying put" and normal routine sometimes violates clique territorial claims in the lounge.

Most mornings, after breakfast, clique members gather in a lounge to read the morning newspaper or chat. Some wheel themselves in and sit near the window. Some walk and move chairs so that they are close enough for conversation. Patients bid each other "good morning" and take up the topic under discussion. The atmosphere is cordial, but it continues to be so only as long as alert patients are present. Normally, various clique members drift in and out of the lounge during this gathering, which lasts for about an hour. By this time, their beds usually have been made and they begin returning to their rooms or go to varied activities on the fifth floor or outdoors.

While clique members gather in a lounge, floor staff goes about its work up and down the hallway. Occasionally, while working in a patient's room, an aide feels that she is being hampered by its occupant. As an aide described, "Some of 'em get in the way so that you can't get your work done." When this happens, and the troublesome patient is not bedridden, the aide may wheel her into the hallway or lounge while "I finish her room." Such patients, however, are usually left where they have been put until all beds have been made.

If a "senile" patient is put in the lounge, it annoys clique members gathered there. The scene is always the same. Members are gathered and quietly chatting when, suddenly, they discover that a person considered senile is on the premises. One member usually whispers vehemently to the others, "Now, why did they have to bring her in here for?" "They" refers to anyone on the floor staff. Other members turn to note the presence of an "obvious" intruder. Witness this episode:

> *Opal Minor (considered senile) sits in her wheelchair, fidgeting with a comb, whining loudly to no one in particular about her husband. The following clique members are gathered: Blanche, Barry, Thelma, Etta, Laura, and Cyrus.*

BLANCHE: How she talks!

BARRY: [To Opal] Stop your whining and talk sense!

> *As the clique members attempt to converse, Opal carries on a stream of talk in which she reacts to single words that she hears in members' conversation. The meanings that Opal gives them are her own. They don't coincide with members' meanings. Opal moans and whines and she talks.*

THELMA: I think they should put them [Senile] on another floor. They shouldn't be with us. They did take three of them to the fourth floor.

BLANCHE: Oh, why doesn't she shut up!

ETTA: Well, she can't help it.

BLANCHE: [Remorsefully] Well, I know it—the poor thing.

LAURA: You don't want to stay in your room and when you come out here, you can't stand it either.

THELMA: They're crazy and they're going to drive you crazy too.

LAURA: That's right.

THELMA: I pay a lot of money in this place and I don't want to listen to that.

BARRY: I don't know why we have to sit here for hours and listen to that crap.

Thelma wheels up to Opal and gives her a lap blanket.

THELMA: [To Opal] You can talk but stop whining because it makes me nervous.

Barry wheels out of the lounge.

LAURA: [To Barry] I don't blame you for leaving. She'll drive us nuts just like she is.

A housekeeping aide walks into the lounge to wash the sink.

CYRUS: [To aide] Jesus, she won't shut up! Why do you all put them in here with us!

AIDE: [Sarcastically] She wants a man to talk to.

CYRUS: [To Opal] Shut up!

All clique members gradually depart, leaving Opal alone in the lounge.

When violations of clique territory occur, members talk of it for some time, in the dining room later in the evening, and in the lounge gathering the next day. Various members of the floor staff also hear of it as clique members pass by and comment on their irresponsibility in "herding everyone together like that."

Clique members are jealous of their ties and work to avoid outsiders on the floor. But at the same time, they pity those whom they consider senile. All agree that ideally one should be humane to all people, no matter how sick. Yet all are practical. They feel that they must make the best of what they have left to live with. To them, this means "keeping people separate." As a clique member put it, "Sure, ya gotta be fair. But, together, it just don't work."

Members guard their ties in other places on the floor. They prefer not to sit at the same dining table with nonmembers. They resent sharing a room with them. They grumble about these and other occasional violations of their ties and protest strongly when the violations are long term.

Connie Wodkowski is a member of an alertness clique. For some time, she shared a room with a woman whom she considered "decent." When it became apparent that her roommate was to be placed in another nursing home, Connie became apprehensive.

Before this roommate arrived, she had shared a room with someone she disliked intensely, and she wondered whether the experience would be repeated.

At the Manor, top staff makes room assignments. They do so
with little or no knowledge of the feelings that the patients on the
floors have about other patients. To top staff, each patient is officially an individual, and each bed, as a place, is separate from
every other one. Certainly, top staff tries to, as it says, "match
patients" in making room assignments. But it does so haphazardly,
its efforts depending on the pressures of administrative work,
psychologistic data on clientele culled from charts, anecdotes,
intake interviews, and the like.

After Connie's roommate left, she considered herself to be the
victim of a very haphazard room assignment indeed. A visibly
dying patient was placed in her room. The patient moaned
around the clock, had large exposed bedsores on her buttocks and
elbows, smelled of decay, and was incontinent. Connie also realized that she "might be stuck with her next to me for some
time." Connie began complaining:

> [To a friend in the dining room] Oh, I can't go into my
> room. You just go in there and see. I've got a very sick
> person in my room. It smells like "corp" [hard "p"] in
> there.

> [To another patient near the nurses' station] You should
> see the sick person they put in my room. And I've got to
> sleep in the same room with her. She was with Miss
> White [member of another clique] before. Miss White
> says that she almost had a nervous breakdown. They have
> a lot of nerve putting that woman with me. I wish my
> sister was here so I could tell her. That's why I'm in my
> wheelchair out here. I'm not going to stay in there.
> Miss White says that she didn't sleep at night at all. She
> nearly drove Miss White crazy.

Connie's complaints grew louder and more hostile the next day.
She refused to cooperate with the floor staff as it did its work.
Several aides reported that Connie had become unusually foul-
mouthed. After another day, the floor staff grew so irritated with
the situation that the charge nurse simply pleaded with her

supervisor for a room change for Connie. Connie was finally moved into Betty White's room. Her protest subsided, but much gossip became attached to the indignity.

Resident Cliques. Cliques on the first floor of the Manor are more varied than on patient floors. The most renowned, the long-time resident clique, becomes known to all persons on the floor soon after they have lived at the Manor for a few days. The entire administrative staff also knows of the clique, often referring to it as the Doherty group, after Mabel Doherty, the very first resident admitted to the Manor.

The Doherty group makes its presence on the first floor felt in several ways. For one thing, it is the only clique in the Manor that has a recognized name. It is part of the public culture of the home. In residents' daily talk about each other, the reference succinctly identifies a group whose members are separate and distinct from others.

Another feature of the clique that maintains its solidarity is talk of the early Manor. When members of the Doherty clique are present in a gathering of residents, references often are made to "what the place was like when it first opened." Members reminisce about the cozy, unrushed atmosphere of the first days of operation. They recall some of the problems that staff faced in starting the home and how they participated directly in early programming for patient care. Margaret Daley, a clique member, once put it this way:

> There were only a few people on this floor when I came. And I must admit, it was a little bit nicer then. It was quieter. And there was less friction. You know how it is. There's a lot of people who come in who are inclined to find fault. Things like that. We were just a kind of family when I came in here. But that couldn't last in an institution like this. They want to make money, you know.

As clique members keep reminding others, the "old days were nicer." To other residents, this signifies that somehow the addition of their presence on the floor has led to its degeneration. They quietly resent this, and more, they resent hearing of it repeatedly.

Not only does the clique associate itself with the golden age of pleasant living on the floor, it knows the Manor's history better than other residents. This makes for conversational presence. In talking about the Manor (of which there is a great deal), all residents may comment on and criticize or praise it in one way or another, but clique members tie their talk to past events. They do it well and, in so doing, often dominate conversation.

When residents and clique members are gathered, talk may be directed to individuals or to the group as a whole. Historical talk, however, has its peculiar style. For example, in talking about the current quality of dining service on the floor, Mabel Doherty turns to another clique member before she details early dining service and says, "You remember when we first came, don't you?" When clique members are present together, detailed, historical talk of the Manor is prefaced by gestures such as nods, sighs, and raised eyebrows that delineate them as residents distinct from others there. Gestures signify their social ties.

The Doherty group is identified with at least two places on the floor. One is the north end of the hallway, where their rooms are located; the other is their table in the dining room. Establishing the table as their place took some time and annoyed several residents in the process.

The clique did not always dine together. Only two members ate at Mabel's table: herself and Pearl Smith. The other two chairs were taken by Homer Wilson and Luis Rodriguez. Homer was a former co-worker of Pearl's at a large department store in town. Homer had shown Luis the "ropes of the place" when Luis first came to the Manor and subsequently was invited to dine at his table.

Mabel was not pleased with this arrangement. She wanted all her good friends to be together. About a month later, Luis was discharged; he entered another nursing home on the west side of town. Mabel saw this as an opportune time to partially close ranks. When residents dined again, she quickly walked to Lenore Wick's table and loudly told her to come and sit with her across the room. Rather awkwardly, Lenore took leave of her table-mates. They felt insulted at what they considered to be the rude departure of someone "who feels we're not good enough for her and her friends." Still later, after Homer died, Mabel succeeded in getting Margaret Daley, the remaining member of her circle, to sit at her table. As one resident scoffed, "Poor Homer's seat was still warm when Margaret moved over there."

Joan Borden makes it quite obvious at times that the Doherty group believes itself to command considerable prestige on the floor. On one occasion, I was having lunch with Joan at her table, together with Martha Cush, another resident. It is common, at table, to offer others food that one isn't going to eat. I asked Joan if she wanted my soda crackers. Before Joan accepted them, she sarcastically shouted, "You better ask Doherty if I can have them first!"

Don Staats described the clique this way:

> There's a couple old crabby bags in there. They hate themselves, I guess. Oh, yeah, there's about three or four old women. Oh, Jesus! When you come walking along, you'd think they're gonna eat you up. Jeez! I don't know what the hell's the matter with 'em, if they just hate themselves or what. I never did anything wrong to 'em. They just look like . . . they're darn ugly! Oh God, they got an awful face on 'em. Oh, man! I feel like givin' 'em a crack in the mouth when I walk by. I feel like I could give 'em a good punch. I call 'em bags. That's all they are. They sit around. . . . You wonder what the hell they're all blabberin' about. Same thing when they're eatin' breakfast or dinner or supper, for God's sake. You wonder how the hell they can shovel the food in their mouth when they got the darn thing open all the time. I guess they're lookin' for a man. Maybe they ain't got any. Maybe the old man croaked away. He couldn't live with 'em Oh, shucks! The hell with it! I got my opinion anyway. I wouldn't let 'em bother me anyway. Good gracious sakes! I don't know what's the matter with 'em. I don't bother 'em at all and they don't bother me. I stay away, far enough away so that I don't have no problems with 'em. Now, why do they gotta get mad at me if I don't talk to them?

The clique has led a fairly successful campaign to ostracize Don. His unwillingness to tolerate what he considers its unreasonable airs and those of other "ladies" on the floor has helped the campaign along.

The first floor has other cliques. Their ties, however, are not as solid and obvious to outsiders as those of the Doherty group. One is the smokers' clique; its ties are sustained by place and resentment. The smokers' clique has three members—Gus Marsh, Cora Mommsen, and Ceil Kukla—who usually gather in the north lounge twice a day to chat and smoke. When they are present there, other residents refrain from sitting in the lounge. If they are about to enter and see the smokers, they often turn and walk away with mild disgust. Many residents, and most of the women, resent smoking. Above all, they resent women smoking. Other cliques on the floor are built around skill at playing particular card games, especially bridge and king's corners.

Friendships

The social ties of clientele within the Manor are not limited to cliques. Each floor has its share of good friends. Friendships differ from cliques in that they are not as concerned as cliques with exclusiveness. Maintaining boundaries is an important thing to clique members, and these boundaries serve to sustain the members' claimed distinction from outsiders. Friends, on the other hand, don't *work* as hard to maintain their ties. They are bound, basically, by tacit sentiment. When asked why they are friends, they are likely to say that they enjoy each other's company or something to that effect. When clique members are asked a similar question, they mention the special basis of their ties in addition to their felt sentiments of attraction.

Two kinds of friendships ties may be distinguished on the floors. Client-to-client friendships are the most common. Client-to-staff friendships occur, also, but these are less common.

Client friendships sometimes have their origins outside the Manor. The migrationlike process by which some clients come to reside at the home means that former acquaintances are likely to reestablish their ties here. Place is also a source of friendship. When asked how they became friends, some clients explain that they met at the dining room table. Others are roommates and have been friends since they began sharing a room. Still others say they met in the lounge, the activity area on the fifth floor, at a religious service on the second floor, or in the first-floor lobby. If patients and residents do not enter the Manor with friends there, do not frequent its public places, and do not have solicitous roommates (or have none at all), they have no friends. There are some clientele like this, and not all are bedridden or nonambulatory. They are the home's social isolates.

Social isolates are considered "strange" by other clientele. No one knows much about them. Their seclusion tends to generate tales about the motives for their isolation, its probable history, and "what they do all by themselves all the time." Social isolates spend most of their time in their rooms, some of them simply sitting and staring into space. They move mostly to perform the most rudimentary tasks of daily living such as voiding, eating, and sleeping. They are not necessarily unintelligible in conversation nor are they great raconteurs.

Like other kinds of social ties, friendship is considered precious by patients and residents. Friends spend much of their social lives together in various places at the Manor—morning until night, most days of the week. Those who are roommates are together around the clock. A change in such ties means a change in their lives. I have witnessed the slightest affront between friends at the Manor result in great personal crises. Until matters between them are resolved, they may feel depressed and frighteningly lonely. Some so totally resign themselves to such lethargy that they make little or no effort to accomplish routines of daily living. When one's world is as small as the floor of a nursing home and its relevant inhabitants are limited to a few friendships, a broken tie may temporarily collapse it all.

The social ties of clientele are ironic in that they are at once so precious and trivial. In the world of patients and residents, ties are cherished. In top staff's world, clientele ties are practically superfluous. In assigning and reassigning clientele rooms, top staff may inadvertently damage or even sever them. For the most part, this is an unwitting consequence of its inadequate knowledge and faulty conception of clientele lives.

Friendship ties between residents and floor staff are rare on the first floor. Those ties that exist on the third and fourth floors typically are between patients and aides. Patients who are bedridden or otherwise relatively dependent on the floor staff may become attached to a particular aide who "is so nice to me." If ties grow, aides give quite generously of their time and services with "their favorites." Rather than perfunctorily completing bed-and-body routines, they spend a good share of their time talking with them and doing a number of favors that they would not otherwise consider part of their jobs.

Aides break any number of official rules for patients with whom they have become friends. At a patient's request, an aide may bring him such items from outside as candy, writing pads, aspirin, laxatives, and cigarettes. Favorites may be allowed to smoke in their rooms behind closed doors under an aide's vigilant eye.

They are allowed to use such staff facilities as telephones at the nurses' station without charge. They may accompany an aide to the employees' lounge on the aide's break. An aide may even surreptitiously take them away from the Manor altogether for a short while on the pretext that they are "just going out in front for a bit." In some ways, having a friend on the staff makes living at the Manor easier than otherwise.

Supporters

A supporter is a person who is socially tied to another by the offer of voluntary assistance. A support tie differs from a clique in that its members are not concerned with exclusiveness. Support differs from friendship in that support is believed to be of some *utility* to the supported, whereas, to be friends, sentiments of mutual attraction are sufficient. These three kinds of ties occur together at times. For example, support may occur between persons who consider themselves good friends.

One of the most typical forms of support at the Manor is help in calling floor staff. Should a patient who needs an aide to help her to the toilet be unable to pull her call buzzer, a roommate may pull it for her. Being a supporter is not a mere social courtesy. Those who consider themselves supporters ("being very good about doing something for someone") expect more than this from themselves. If an aide does not come after she is buzzed, a supporter proceeds to engage one in some way. She may walk down the hallway and ask the help of an aide who passes by. She may even go to the nurses' station and request help.

Some supporters complete their tasks rather dramatically. Take Bertha Thomas, for instance, a wheelchair patient on the third floor. Bertha is considered "sharp as a tack" by the floor staff and is a member of an alertness clique. Bertha is concerned for the care of those patients whom she considers "sad and not able to do for themselves" and makes it her business to see that the staff "treats them right."

On one occasion, Sarah Bushnell is seated restrained in a wheelchair near the nurses' station. Bertha is chatting with another patient nearby. Sarah tries to rise from her chair but slips to one side as the restraint tugs at her. Bertha sees this and notices that the nurses at the station are doing nothing to help her. She courteously asks the nurses to attend Sarah. When this has no effect, Bertha becomes furious. And right in the middle of the hallway, she screams at the top of her lungs, "Nurse! Help!" This startles the nurses. Bertha then calmly tells them to attend to Sarah, which they do.

Many other forms of support tie clientele to each other. Some ambulatory patients consistently push wheelchair patients to desired locations. This is quite evident as patients leave the dining area for their own rooms or when a wheelchair patient's destination is "way down the hallway" or on some other floor. Some patients who are unsteady on their feet link arms when they walk. This steadies them both. It is quite common for patients to take walks arm-in-arm even though they are mere acquaintances. Other patients consistently volunteer to read letters, bills, and postcards to those with poor eyesight. It is not unusual for those with "good eyes" to be widely known on a floor as the "ones you see if you want to know what it says." A few clients even develop mutually supportive ties. I first learned that two residents were habitual eyes and ears for each other when I was sitting in the Manor's lounge one day. As they sat down to wait for lunch, one said to the other, "Sit here and listen for the trays. You can hear them better than I can. Then I'll read this letter for you."

Interfloor Ties

A number of patients and residents maintain social ties between floors. Some of these ties even existed before the persons involved became residents of the Manor. An ambulatory person may visit a former friend who is bedridden on a different floor. Typically, this leads to a periodic "visit upstairs" to renew acquaintance or to play cards, bingo, and the like. In a few cases, relatives reside on different floors of the Manor. Currently, two male residents have spouses on the third floor whom they visit several times daily.

Some interfloor ties result from clientele moves from one floor to another. If a resident grows ill or has an accident, he may be moved to a patient floor, where nursing personnel are most readily available. Transferred residents maintain ties with friends on the first floor primarily through visits. If they subsequently regain residential status, they sometimes visit acquaintances they made while patients on the third or fourth floor.

Interfloor moves are made for other reasons than illness. If there is a question about the care status of an incoming individual, he is likely to be placed on a higher floor. "Mistakes" in assignments sometimes lead to subsequent moves. Relatives of a resident or patient may request that he be moved to another floor. "Unruly" residents may be transferred upstairs. When new wings or floors are opened, clientele are sometimes shifted from one to another. All of these elaborate the interfloor ties of clientele.

Certain public places in the Manor generate and/or sustain interfloor ties. These include the chapel on the second floor, the activity area on the fifth floor, the beauty and barber shop on the third floor, the physical therapy area on the fourth floor, and the home's grounds. A few residents and patients who consider themselves alert prefer to visit each other in such public places rather than in conventional patient areas. To them, this means "a nicer visit since not so many of the senile ones are around."

Finally, some interfloor ties are maintained through third parties. Periodic shifts in the floor assignment of aides and nurses make it possible for members of the floor staff to serve as links between clientele on different floors. Outsiders such as relatives and friends of clientele on different floors serve the same function.

All in all, the social ties of clientele are more complex than top staff cares to imagine. It often wonders, though, how its "secrets" so quickly become public knowledge among patients and residents. And it is sometimes puzzled by the "strange" products of the social relations among clientele, such as their persistent social obligations and avoidances.

CONCLUSION

In Chapter 2, I tried to show how top staff officially conceives of the social world of clientele. To top staff, the clientele world is peopled by individuals who allegedly need nursing home services and who respond to the individualized, total care that floor staff provides them. This conception is simplistic in that it largely ignores the complexities of the social relations among clientele and the social conventions and obligations that arise with such complexities. However, as I have documented in this chapter, the varied dimensions of clientele social relations are indeed more complex than top staff's official conception supposes them to be.

For the most part, top staff is insulated from the ongoing complexities that exist within the social world of clientele. This is largely a matter of place. Top staff gains "information" about clientele and makes decisions about it in places other than those in which clientele maintain their social ties. Likewise, clientele do not enter those places in which top staff makes decisions about them in its highly psychologistic fashion.

In the next chapter, I turn to another social world, that of the floor staff, which lies between those of top staff and clientele. A good part of what is done here "rectifies" for clientele events occurring in the world of top staff and vice versa. Again, this is done in certain places, often insulated from either top staff or clientele.

Bed-
and-
Body
Work

The routine work of nurses and aides on the floors is situated between the worlds of top staff and clientele. The work is routine in the sense that its members guard its regularity and resent any innovations. When top staff issues directives aimed at changing some features of patient care, floor staff responds in such a way as to give "sufficient" evidence of having complied while minimizing change in what "it always does with these people."

Floor staff is wary as well about sources of change within the world of patients and resident. Clientele have various resources by which to influence floor staff's work, ranging from uncooperativeness to complaining to relatives or top staff about what they consider inappropriate treatment. Nurses and aides on the floor know of these resources and know those who are most adept at using them. Their conservatism leads them to avoid possible sources of change in the world of clientele or to routinize the "annoyances" if they do occur.

On the whole, floor staff is fairly successful at maintaining normal work routines. This, however, involves a good deal of work. It means that members of the floor staff must learn to be proficient at dealing with "annoyances" of both superiors and clientele. Most do. Although some member of the floor staff may occasionally refuse to or hasn't yet "learned the ropes," she eventually learns to comply with floor standards since her integration into the floor's work life depends on it.

BED-AND-BODY WORK

Normal work routine is primarily a matter of bed-and-body work. In practice, floor staff believes that once beds have been made and the highly visible bodily needs of clientele have been attended to, it has accomplished a day's work. It becomes "fed up," as its members say, when anything interferes with this. Floor staff pays lip service to ideals that approximate top staff's conception of total patient care, but what it attends to on the floors and grumbles about as it conducts its business is bed-and-body work. Rarely does floor staff become as obviously irritated with the lack of total patient care on the floors as it does with an occasional lapse of normal bed-and-body routine.

Regardless of work shift, the content of bed-and-body routine is the same. What varies is its sequencing and the proportions of its components. On one shift, bed work occurs early; on another shift, it occurs later. The same is true of body work. On one shift, the amount of body work may be about the same as bed work; on another, work is mostly a matter of attending to the bodily needs of patients and residents.

Floor staff does not merely make sure that clientele get through the stages of everyday living, such as awakening, eating, and sleeping; it prepares them to enter each stage as well. Many patients simply cannot make good on their awareness that it is time to accomplish one routine or another.

The regularity of clientele life in nursing homes is similar to that of clientele in other total institutions such as prisons and mental hospitals.[1] In each, staff is actively involved in scheduling daily living. However, scheduling is not the same as accomplishing. In many total institutions with internal clientele and staffs, clientele are believed capable of accomplishing scheduled routines, but this is not so in nursing homes. Floor staffs in nursing homes, for example, virtually do some clientele's eating and voiding *with* them.

[1] See Erving Goffman, *Asylums* (New York: Doubleday, 1961).

Awakening

The daily life of clientele begins with awakening. Because floor staff must wake some patients, awakening begins very early in the morning. The fewer the number of aides present on the floors the earlier it is. As one aide explained,

> It depends on how many aides you have on the floor. One place I worked, I was the only one on the ward. I had to start getting them up at four-thirty. It just takes time to get them ready. Sometimes you even have to wash them up *after* breakfast. You just don't have the time.

At the Manor, even with what is considered to be a full complement of aides (eight to ten per floor), awakening is considered part of the night shift's work. The night shift, which leaves work at 7:30 A.M., typically begins to awaken patients at about 5:30 A.M. When the time is ready, aides walk down the hall and notify everyone that it is "time to wake up." How they do this depends on aides' conceptions of the "trouble" patients are likely to make if "you wake them up too early or too late" or too abruptly.

In order to have everyone ready for breakfast at approximately the same time with minimal disturbance to normal routine, aides usually sequence awakening. Patients who must be taken to the dining room but who require extensive help in getting ready are awakened first. Those whom floor staff considers alert, self-helping, and apt to complain are awakened last. Also awakened later are bed patients known as "feeders." They have their meals in bed and must be fed by the aides. A few may even have to be helped to swallow their food and drink. Sequencing takes place throughout the day before each meal. As one aide said:

> The night shift starts getting them up at five-thirty. Where I worked at other nursing homes, they did the same. I guess most nursing homes get the patients up then. We don't get all the patients up at the same time though. Those who get up easy, we get up first. Some like to sleep longer. We just tell them to get up and then come back for them later.

When aides make mistakes and get the "wrong patients up and ready too early," they are likely to hear of it soon and quite plainly. As Louise Kramer, a fourth-floor patient, reports:

I just don't understand why the aides wheel the patients down to the dining room so early. They wake us up with a hurry-hurry attitude. They take us in the dining room and we sit! I've sat there for as much as an hour and a half. One time I got so mad after breakfast when they left me here for an hour that I just screamed loud at them. They came up to me and said, "We don't do that here, Louise." I thought, "Well, if I can't move, at least I can scream."

Aides also try to avoid invading the privacy of those patients and residents who are known to be very sensitive about it, since they, too, can make trouble for normal routine on the floor. As one aide stated:

Some of them, like Blanche and Mrs. Wayne . . . they like their privacy. We just knock on their doors and they usually answer back that they heard. The others, especially those who always have their call light pulled, we just walk in on them and wake them up.

Aides on the night shift see to it that most patients and residents are at least awake and dressing before the next shift comes to work. When they are slack, newly arriving aides become angry. The floor staff on the day shift considers it the duty of the night shift to have clientele nearly ready for breakfast. When they are not, day aides and nurses yell at night aides about all manner of things: "Now, we're going to have complaints all day about late breakfast!" "How are we going to do our treatments and meds, and get everyone ready too!" "This is going to be one of those days." "We're not going to get anything done today and we'll catch hell for it too." "Sure it's easy for you, but do you know what kind of goddamn day that means for us!"

Body Work

Bed-and-body work begins immediately upon awakening. Incontinent patients usually are changed after they are awakened. If this is "one of those days" when aides feel rushed, they may take patients to the dining room wet or soiled. This may be hidden easily by wheelchairs, lap blankets, or robes, or it may be accounted for by stating that the particular patient involved "voided" or "must have had a BM after I got him ready." Or he may be said to be a "soaker," one of those patients about whom "you can never tell when they'll let loose."

The body work in getting clientele ready for the day varies widely. Among residents and some patients, aides are not involved at all. As a matter of fact, such clientele resent interference by aides in their daily ablutions. As floor staff says, "You learn who you have to leave alone."

With other clientele, especially those patients whom one aide called "heavies," body work is a very intimate affair. Aides must move them limb by limb in order to do their work. Such patients are helpless in performing the variety of basic daily functions for themselves. The very heaviest of these are bedfast patients. They commonly wear urinary catheters. Although this saves aides the work of changing wet beds and clothing, it does not rid them of the labor of cleaning the products of a bowel movement.

The speech of some helpless patients is unintelligible. Aides consider working with them to be like dealing with "big babies." One aide said: "They can't tell you what they want or if something hurts. You have to second-guess everything for them. And they still need everything that everyone else does. They gotta eat and sleep the same. They're helpless . . . like babies, but bigger."

Dealing with such patients often takes two aides. These patients have to be turned periodically to slow the development of bedsores; they have to be given bed baths; they must be fed. All this has to be completed without the cooperation of the patient.

In dealing with "heavies," aides expect to give help to each other and to receive such help. Any aide may be assigned these patients, and thus stands the chance of needing help. When one has to work on the body of a heavy patient, she solicits another's assistance. For the most part, help is offered readily. The two exceptions to this are when an aide has not yet learned of this informal mutual assistance rule, and when an aide is consistently unwilling to help others with such patients. Eventually, an uncooperative aide is neither sought for nor given help. These aides are considered "hard to work with."

Soiled, heavy patients are often changed without being taken from bed. Two aides usually are needed for this. Both roll the patient to one side; then one holds the patient steady while the other replaces or adjusts bedding on the other side. This is repeated by rolling the patient the other way. Bed patients who regularly use the toilet in their rooms must be lifted from their beds and helped there. This too can be a job requiring two aides.

In working with "heavies," aides sometimes make use of a Hoyer lifter, a cranelike device that mechanically lifts a patient with an arm and leg sling. Aides are taught to use this device at in-service classes. Although it is said that with the lifter and proper technique an aide "should be able to care for any patient alone," in practice, aides do not care for all patients alone. Although most appreciate various devices like the lifter and patient care techniques taught at in-service, floor work is treated as a more practical affair.

Bed-and-body work is always considered to be rushed. Floor staff frequently complains that "there's just no time to do everything." This sentiment translates into the belief that one simply cannot do everything "by the book." As one aide said, "You do the best you can in the time you have and that means doing it your way." Devices and equipment that "are used in modern patient care," like the Hoyer lifter, may not be available at the time or place they are needed. Rather than conduct a search for equipment, aides tend to improvise. This often means teamwork.

The informal mutual assistance rule does not extend to all bed-and-body work. It is confined mostly to work with heavy patients, and occasionally to work with unruly ones. Otherwise, aides are expected to do their own work. When someone does not, others grumble, complain among themselves, and sometimes "tell her off." Each aide considers her patient load "heavy enough as it is without having to do someone else's crap too." Thus, when one aide solicits help from another, she usually makes it clear that help is necessary.

The clarity of an aide's need for help influences whether or not she is considered to be "carrying her share of the work around here." When other aides are asked to help for what they feel "is no good reason at all," they become irritated since it keeps them from "normally" completing their own routines. Most aides are aware of the tacit conditions under which help is appropriately solicited. They know when to invoke the need for help and when not to.

Obstacles to Bed-and-Body Work

When patients are considered ready, those who must be taken to the dining room are wheeled there; those who can make it on their own, either by walking or wheeling, do so. Those patients who "dillydally," as the aides say, are hurried along with the others. Feeders remain in their rooms, where their trays are brought by the aide assigned to them.

Floor staff is often quite glib about what those patients and residents who ready themselves for various events of the day "do in their rooms." Aides see themselves as being rushed but at the same time efficiently accomplishing bed-and-body work on the floor. They feel that self-help clientele, especially on patient floors, do "a lot of foolin' around before they get anything done." To aides, "foolin' around" is useless activity that tends to slow down normal floor routine. Because aides consider it both useless to the patients themselves and an impediment to their own work, they easily dismiss it as nothing to be considered seriously.

There is a certain degree of moral indignation in aides' attitudes toward patients' "foolin' around." After all, as one aide said, "Here we are workin' our tails off for them. Do you think I have time to deal and wait for all their fartin' around? Sometimes, you just gotta get 'em goin'."

Aides believe that the fact they're working for the patients, and working hard at that, is good enough reason to "get 'em goin'." Thus, aides may enter rooms and urge patients along to their scheduled destinations with obvious exasperation or patronizing indulgence. Typical statements on these occasions express their sentiments: "What *are* we going to do with you, Cora?" "What, for God's sake, could be so important about all this? Let's get moving now." "Look! I've got a lot of work to do. I can't wait for you to finish all this silly stuff." Or an aide may say to another one in reference to patients' "foolin' around": "What are we going to ever do with these people?" "You know how she has to take her fucking time about everything and do everything just so-so. If I don't get her out of there, she'll never eat." "Oh well. [Sighs] Patients are patients."

Aides take patients to the dining room three times a day. Breakfast necessitates the most extensive bed-and-body work, since many patients must be awakened and dressed before the meal. Some premeal events slow down bed-and-body work. For example, patients may insist on being taken to toilet or having the bedpan when an aide is ready to take them to the dining room for lunch or supper. Or someone may soil his clothing in such a way that it is difficult to hide from anyone or pass off as unnoticed.

Once patients are in the dining room, food is not served immediately. Typically, those patients who have been taken there first because "they're not complainers" sit in their wheelchairs or regular chairs at the table for some time. They wait through two premeal events before they eat. First, they wait through the time it takes the floor staff to get all patients who are scheduled to eat in the dining room seated there. This ranges anywhere from a half-hour to a full hour. Second, they wait for their food trays to arrive from the kitchen. This is usually later than what the floor staff considers to be the scheduled time to eat. Altogether, some patients may wait seated in the dining room for up to an hour and a half before their food is placed in front of them.

For the most part, dining room waiting by patients does not lead to disruption of floor staff's normal work routine. Aides are fairly successful at sequencing patients in such a way that "you don't hear any complaints from 'em." However, this doesn't mean that those who don't complain are satisfied with the situation. Many are not. A good part of talk among themselves deals with what they consider the inordinate amount of waiting they often endure.

Occasionally, a patient or resident who has been left waiting for what he believes is too long a period of time "makes trouble" for the floor staff. "Making trouble" may mean screaming in rage about undue waiting. Sometimes it means throwing dishes or trays on the floor. Or it may mean wheeling or walking about in anger. Whatever form it takes, "making trouble" disrupts what the floor staff believes to be normal routine.

When floor staff describes patients who "make trouble," it uses the language employed by top staff to talk about what the latter considers the problematic behavior of individual residents or patients. For example, a person who screams in rage at waiting for his food may be said to be *disoriented*. One who throws dishes or walks about in anger is *agitated* or *confused*. On the face of it, this language locates the source of clientele problems in their personal actions. It suggests that something is wrong with the resident or patient, not with the situation in which he is involved. The language is used by floor staff mostly in reference to clientele who disrupt what it believes to be normal work routines.

Although both floor and top staff describe problematic clientele in the same language, what they do to alleviate their problems differs. Top staff writes individually-oriented care plans or issues similar directives (memos) to the floor staff. To top staff, one gets rid of patient problems by treating the individual patient or resident. Floor staff is more likely to deal with the situation that generates the problem. It may try to accommodate its routine treatment of clientele in such a way that they have no reason to "make trouble." For example, it tries to shorten the wait of "complainers." Or it may routinize annoyances in ways that prevent clientele from disrupting normal work routine. For example, it may temporarily sequester patients who "make trouble" in certain situations by wheeling them into the far corner of a distant room.

Dining

There is fairly wide variation in the ways clientele eat at the Manor, ranging from the genteel dining of residents to helping certain patients to eat.

Residents' Dining Room. Residents expect their dining to be gracious. The three daily meals they have at the Manor are times when they are most visible to the resident population as a whole. On these occasions, it is important to appear to be and be treated as "normal, competent" elders.

The physical setting of the first-floor dining room is different from that of patient dining areas. It is located in what is the south lounge area on other floors. The room is smaller than patient dining rooms. It is carpeted, has dim lighting, and is partially paneled with wood, creating a mood that is warmer and more sober than other dining areas at the Manor.

The mood of this dining room pervades the behavior of those who occupy it. Residents enter the premises decorously. They walk to and seat themselves at tables with as much composure as they can manage. Once there, they exchange greetings and engage in subdued conversation with tablemates. The weather is often discussed briefly. Anyone who publicly deviates from this routine can expect to receive annoyed frowns and irritated sighs from the others present.

Usually, two members of the floor staff work in the first-floor dining area. One is the hostess who at other times sits behind the nurses' station; she distributes trays to residents. The other is an RN or LPN who distributes medications. Residents expect the hostess and medication nurse to treat them as normal, adult patrons of the room. Floor staff is quite aware of this. To avoid trouble, it usually accommodates residents' wishes, but it resents doing so because it makes them feel subservient to the residents. As one aide complained, "You just feel like a waitress." But to most members of the floor staff who "work the floor," momentary resentment is "easier to live with than a lot of complaining old biddies."

Trays arrive from the kitchen on a large swivel cart. The hostess carefully places each tray in front of a resident. She avoids being too abrupt. When all trays are distributed, she begins pouring coffee, tea, or whatever beverage residents are accustomed to drinking. Should some item on a resident's tray be missing, the hostess obtains it. Throughout the meal, she is at the service of diners.

While residents eat, the medication nurse distributes medications. This is a delicate procedure since the mood of the place is supposedly one of "normal" adult living, or as nearly "normal" as participants can make it given their tacit but persistent awareness that they indeed reside in a nursing home. To sustain this mood, the nurse puts pills and liquids in small paper cups and discreetly places them next to the appropriate person's plate. She then quietly goes on with the rest of her business.

On those occasions when floor staff is not appropriately subservient, it is roundly castigated by residents. Sometimes this means a harsh complaint to the top staff about the transgression; sometimes it means an immediate, embarrassing insult. When the floor staff member involved is repeatedly "uppity" or "rude," residents have been known to spread vicious rumors about her. This usually involves deliberate indiscretions in her presence, such as carrying on a presumably private conversation about her that is just loud enough for her to overhear. One aide's experience as hostess was reported this way:

> Mr. Swanson [a resident who later became a patient] thinks he's just so-so, but I think he's a goddamn bastard. You shoulda seen how he treated me when I used to serve in the dining room on one. One time, when I was pouring his coffee, he asked me to pour only a quarter cup. Well, so I happened to go a bit higher. So he gets pissed and tells me that I oughtta do things right because I'd always be an aide since I don't have much education. Can you believe that? Then he tells me that he's quite educated

and that I should respect him. Well, Jesus! I got really mad, but I didn't show it. I picked up his cup, poured it out, and poured his damn quarter cup for him. So then he gets insulted and mutters, "bitch," under his breath. I prefer working up here on three. Those people down there are just too demanding. They think we're here just to wait on them. They treat us like dirt.

Patients' Dining Rooms. On the whole, the atmosphere of patient dining rooms is more impersonal and rushed than the residents' dining room. When trays arrive, they are often dropped in front of patients. This annoys those who feel they are "really like residents except that we've been put up here." Alertness cliques on patient floors never cease to talk about the "treatment we get from some of these aides." Sounds of clacking dishes and loud talk between aides is common: "Where's Stella's tray?" "Mary, get Helen a fork!" "Who's going to pick up that broken glass?"

Aides are less subservient to patients than they are to residents. They "herd" patients through their meals. When patients indicate that they aren't going to finish some part of their meals, aides typically comment on it, and loudly too: "Aren't you going to finish your chicken?" "You didn't clean your plate." "Now Lucille. Let's eat that all up!" This very rarely occurs on the first floor, where what a resident eats and what he doesn't is considered his own business for the most part.

Aides often coax patients to eat something that they consider beneficial to the patient or that they believe the patient likes. They are curt and condescending to those they believe "don't know what they're doing anyway." Joe Maas, for instance, has a poor appetite and often leaves much of his meal uneaten. When he's consumed what he wants, he leaves the table and returns to his room. This annoys Barbara Kemp, an aide on the floor who claims to know what's best for Joe. On one occasion, similar to many others, Joe begins to move his chair in the process of leaving the table. From across the room, Barbara notices this because, as she says, "I keep my eye on him." She shouts at him, "Joe! Sit down!" Rushing to this table, she takes his fork and begins hacking and virtually smashing his peaches. She then picks up a bit of the peachy mess, brings it to his mouth, nudging his closed lips, and exclaims: "Here! Eat! Sweet! You like sweet! So eat this!" Her sentences indicate that she considers that she is talking to someone not fully rational. Joe leaves the table abruptly.

Patients who are prone to dribble their food on the floor or their clothing are "bibbed." Some of them must be fed. This process can be quite untidy as food is spilled on the table and on both patient and aide. Between mouthfuls, aides often wipe patients' chins and faces. Occasionally, a patient urinates or defecates while he or she is dining. As long as this isn't too obvious, feeding is completed before a change in clothing is made. While sneezing or coughing, patients may smear mucus on themselves, their plates, and aides as they awkwardly reach for various items on their trays and simultaneously try to maintain their composure. To floor staff, cleaning up such patients is all part of normal body work with some people on the third and fourth floors of the Manor.

When "alert" patients desire something that has not been placed on their trays, aides are likely to improvise before they call for it or go to the kitchen to get it. They may slyly look around at what's available on the trays of those patients whom they "know" are senile or won't "make trouble." If they find what is needed, they'll take it and discreetly offer it to a "complainer." After all, as they claim, "We just don't have the time to go through all that. You just make do."

After they are finished eating, patients are sequenced out of the dining room—those apt to "make trouble" first, and so on. Again, the nonambulatory, noncomplainers wait. Emptying the room sometimes takes a whole hour.

Treatments

Medications are distributed and treatments done several times a day. This is the work of RNs and LPNs on the floor staff. On the first floor, residents' medications are distributed mostly at mealtime. On patient floors, treatments are more common than among residents. They are done, along with the distribution of "meds," in the morning, afternoon, and evening after patients return to their rooms from the dining area.

Treatments include such things as changing bandages, cleaning open wounds with hydrogen peroxide, applying skin salves, and the like. One of the floor nurses does half the hallway and another does the other half. A cart containing a variety of medical supplies and prescribed medications is wheeled from room to room. Patients are accustomed to this routine and treat it as a normal part of daily life at the Manor. As with other phases of bed-and-body work, their day is partially structured by it. Every morning, afternoon, and evening, some time after eating, patients expect to receive a personal visit from one of the nurses on the floor. They are usually in or near their rooms at this time.

To floor nurses, a treatment is regular and orderly when everyone involved is at least superficially pleasant. Typically, this means that when a nurse enters a patient's room to do a treatment or administer "meds," there is, first, an exchange that pokes fun at the regularity of her visits. A nurse may say: "Here we go again, George." "Another treatment, Mrs. Kramer." "It's that time again." Or a patient may comment in jest: "Oh, it's you again." "Will I ever get rid of you, Miss Renska?" "Another day, another salve job."

When treatments are being performed, normal body routine involves a "positive attitude" by both nurse and patient about what is taking place. Patients are expected to act at least mildly cheerful when being treated, no matter how apparently hopeless their condition. Nurses expect the same of themselves. For example, Sally Martin (an LPN) enters June Burton's room. After a few pleasantries, Sally hands June her pills, which are round and brown. June turns to Sally and scoffs, as she does daily, "Mouse turds again!" Sally, as she also does daily, laughs briefly. When a patient is morbid or cynical about his or her own physical condition, the nurse quickly points out the "positive side" of things. A routine treatment is one that is completed with minimal social effort. Take June Burton again. Sally Martin is about to begin her leg treatments by applying pressured oxygen to them. June's legs are crossed while she waits in her wheelchair. As Sally proceeds to uncross her legs, June moans and gives a small scream. Sally lowers the right leg to the floor. June exclaims, "Oh, I wish they'd take an ax and cut this leg off. This shouldn't happen to ninety-eight-year-old woman." Sally answers, "What do you mean? Aren't you queen bee around here?" Sally refers to June's being crowned "Queen" on Grandparent's Day for being the oldest female at the Manor. June answers, "Do you think it's fun to be real old? You all should open your eyes. People should die before they get to be like me. Old age is no fun!" As Sally gets ready to move on, she glibly pleads, "Aw, come on, Mrs. Burton. You shouldn't think like that." Sally walks out.

Although aides don't treat patients, they are witness to and come into direct contact with their physical states. For the most part, they routinize the care of what, in another context, might be considered repugnant. Occasionally, however, it becomes known that there is a case of extreme physical deterioration on one of the floors. As one aide stated to another, "Have you seen Alice Wilson's foot lately? It's so rotten that when you lift it up, the bone falls out." Being curious, some aides deliberately "come down" or "come up" to the floor "to see what it's like." They all act momentarily shocked and pass on the word about "how bad it is." On subsequent days, as the news spreads, other aides "take a look." The condition of the foot becomes part of the routine talk about work in which floor staff members engage among themselves.

Bed-making

A considerable part of bed-and-body work is devoted to making beds. This is aide work. All members of the floor staff know that neatly made beds are, to their superiors, one of the prime indicators that patients are being properly attended. Aides are vigilant about this.

Bed-making is a ritualized affair. Part of this, of course, is due to state requirements about bedding in nursing homes. Certain types of sheets must be used. Some must be placed under or over others. Some kinds of materials cannot legally come into contact with clientele. But aside from this, aides recognize and invidiously compare poorly made beds with well-made beds. Well-made ones are smooth, properly and tightly tucked at the bottom, and covered by the spread so that top sheets don't visibly droop out the sides. Above all, a well-made bed is tightly made. This means that bottom tucks are *secure* and top sheets *taut*. Indeed, the criterion for well-made beds is met so well by a few aides that some patients occasionally have difficulty getting into bed.

Once beds are made, aides try to keep them made as long as possible. To remake a bed "just slows us down." When clientele desire to take a nap, they are discouraged from "mussing it up too much." They are told to lie *on* the bed, not in it. When they do climb into it, aides become irritated and complain bitterly:

"Now you messed that up again!" "What are you doing in bed?" "Now I'm going to have to fix that bed all over again!"

Although most patients are aware of floor staff's desire to keep beds made and rooms neat, they sometimes also want to take a nap. This poses a dilemma for those who wish to avoid disrupting normal floor routine.

On one occasion, a patient on the fourth floor, Maria Rupini, is "aching for some sleep." She walks to the nurses' station and asks to see the nurse. An LPN asks her what she wants. In a quiet pleading voice, Maria says,

> Can I go to sleep? When I sleep on my bed, that's the only way I get relief. The girl [aide] in my room was making my bed and she said not to lay down on it. But that's the only way I get relief from this pain.

The nurse tells Maria that she can go to her room and lie down if she wishes. Maria asks, "Should I tell the girl that?" The nurse answers, "Yes." Then Maria remembers that she feels cold but the aide who made her bed doesn't want her to use the covers. Maria tells this to another aide, who subsequently gets her a small lap blanket. Maria is satisfied and walks to her room.

Toileting

Toileting and bowel work is another feature of bed-and-body routines. Toileting is a staff word that refers to helping patients void. Bowel work includes giving laxatives and enemas, removing bowel impactions, rinsing stool from patients' clothing and bedding, cleaning bedpans, cleansing patients of fecal matter that may have been smeared on their bodies, keeping track of the frequency and texture of bowel movements, and keeping rooms free from odors.

Aides use a variety of techniques to expedite bowel work. For example, an aide who finds that one of her patients has somehow smeared stool over much of his clothing and body is not likely to painstakingly "clean it all bit by bit." Rather, she virtually "hoses him down." As one aide described it: "We strip 'em bare. Then we get the shower chair and put 'em in it. Then we wheel 'em down the hall to the shower and hose 'em down."

Or take this contingency. A third-floor patient who spends much of her time in bed requested a bedpan. The aide placed it

under her and left. It was about time to take patients to the
dining room. The aide returned a while later and told the patient
that she was "going to take her down the hall for lunch." The
patient objected because she was not finished and, in addition,
claimed to have diarrhea. Feeling rushed, the aide then said that
the patient could ride down to lunch sitting on her bedpan and
that "no one would notice because we'll wrap a lap blanket
around you." Although this may have resolved this bowel contingency for the aide in other cases, it did not in this one. As the
patient said later.

> She even wanted to take me to the dining room while I
> had diarrhea. I told her I wasn't going because I had to
> be on the bedpan. She said that I didn't have diarrhea
> because it was soupy and mine wasn't. I told her that
> I've had this for the last six months and that I should
> know what diarrhea looks like. Well, then, she said that
> she'd put me on my wheelchair on the bedpan with a
> blanket over it and that no one would notice. Have you
> ever heard of such nerve! I don't care if no one would
> notice. *I'd* know I was on it! And what about the odor?

In order to minimize the disruptions in routine bed-and-body
work that untoileted bowel movements can cause, some aides
make a practice of trying to second-guess bowel accidents. When
they "spot certain patients moving around in a funny way," they
consider it time to toilet them. As these aides would say, "You
can just tell. That's all." Occasionally, one aide will inform another that she has just "spotted" a patient assigned to the latter
who looks like he or she needs toileting. When "spotted" patients
do not have bowel movements during toileting, aides become
vexed and conclude that the patient "is just holding it."

Whenever patients (but not residents) have a bowel movement, aides record it in a defecation book. It is the Manor's own
policy and presumably is used as a means of communication
about patients' bowels from one shift to another. The book contains what are called BM lists. These are weekly tallies of the
frequency and texture of patients' movements. Frequency on each
shift is recorded by number. Texture is coded: N: normal stool;
D: diarrhea; CS: constipated stool (hard and small). Some aides
add further descriptions of their own such as quantity (large or
small), whether or not it looks "normal," presence of flatus,

"gone" indicating flushed away before inspection), and impaction.

In practice, entries to the book are made haphazardly. New aides tend to keep bowel records, but veterans ignore them for the most part. Contrary to top staff's belief, the book is rarely used for intershift communication. As it turns out, each shift deals pretty much with the problems it faces on its own shift. Aides do not like to complete "work that was last shift's job."

The defecation book is often buried among other pamphlets and papers at the nurses' station. On those rare occasions when someone is searching seriously for it, most aides don't readily know where to find it. When I looked for it myself, I was often asked, "Why are you interested in *that?* We don't really use it, you know." Inspection of its contents makes that obvious.

A good deal of bowel talk goes on between aides on any one shift. This talk is quite routine, for it's work talk. For example, one aide may be sitting at the nurses' station when another approaches and pauses for a moment. In making conversation, the one sitting mentions, "Frank had a BM today." The other aide answers, "Oh yeah? That's good." The first aide concludes, "It was kinda grayish white."

Bowel work and talk is part of Manor routine. When bowel work is particularly disgusting, floor personnel are disgusted. Although it is an integral part of bed-and-body work, nurses and aides take "little precautions" to make bowel work less obnoxious. Some handle stool delicately. Some try to avoid continual eye contact with it, preferring to "look just enough to know what you're doing." A few even defend themselves with perfume. "I didn't put my perfume on today. When I work upstairs [patient floors], I have the habit of putting perfume on my tits so that when I have to step over to clean, I smell the perfume and not the BM."

Bathing

All clientele are scheduled for weekly baths. Residents see to this themselves. On patient floors, however, aides treat bathing as they do dining. This means that when they consider it time for patients to take baths, it is done in as expeditious and orderly a manner as possible. Complainers are left to the end of bath schedules when "there's more time to handle 'em." The "easy ones" are done when things are more rushed.

Institutional Plain

The perfunctory bathing and dressing involved in bed-and-body work homogenizes the appearance of aide-dependent patients. After living at the Manor for a while, women come to be dressed and coiffured in "institutional plain." Routine body work does not typically lend itself to carefully matching apparel, seeing that clothes and hairstyling suit a patient's personal taste, applying cosmetics, caring for dentures, or paying attention to such accessories as bracelets, earrings and the like. This means that aide-dependent patients are likely to appear tastelessly dressed, wan, uncombed, gray, and toothless.

As with other aspects of their work on the floor, aides and nurses become accustomed to the routine appearance of clientele. "Institutional plain" is treated as the normal mien of some patients. Floor staff gives little thought to it, except on certain rare occasions. If a "plain" female patient is taken to the beauty shop to have her hair styled, aides are genuinely amazed when she returns to the floor. They are likely to comment that they "just can't believe it." For the moment, it becomes a spectacle over which they urge each other, from one end of the hall to the other, to "go and take a look." A day or two later, appearance returns to normal.

Another event that amazes the routine-prone floor staff is being shown pre-Manor photos of "plain" patients. Sometimes a relative and occasionally the patient himself share such pictures with aides and nurses on the floor. As with an unusual coif, floor staff looks, is surprised, and gossips about it. Again, as one aide said, "You just can't believe that that's the same person that's here."

Time Use

Floor staff resents the intrusion of bed-and-body work on its official free time at the Manor. When it is time for members of the floor staff to take a break or eat, they usually are eager to leave. For example, Minnie Sealy, a fourth-floor patient who's sitting in her wheelchair next to the nurses' station says, "I've got to go to the toilet." Diane Wilkens, an aide who is about to leave for lunch answers, "Just a minute, Minnie." Diane looks for another aide. When Pam Koski walks by, Diane asks, "Will you take Minnie to the toilet before she drives us all crazy?" Pam, who is just about ready to leave for lunch herself, reluctantly takes Minnie and puts her on the toilet. Pam then leaves for lunch and says,

"She can sit on the toilet by herself. When she's done, she'll pull the buzzer." Five minutes later, Minnie's buzzer sounds. An aide hears it and calls to another aide, "I can't get that because I have to go. Darlene, it's all yours.'

At shift change, work personnel overlap for a half-hour. Presumably, this time is used to pass information about patient care on one shift to the next. This is mostly a charge-nurse–to–charge-nurse exchange. Aides on both shifts, on the other hand, mill about the nurses' station, creating a partylike atmosphere. There is much bantering, and they laugh and tease each other. Patients are ignored momentarily; charting is completed flippantly; bed-and-body work is forgotten. It all can wait for a few minutes.

Patients and residents begin to retire about 7 P.M. For residents, this is a personal matter. Some patients, on the other hand, are put to bed. For the most part, the task is completed by 9 P.M. By then, all is fairly quiet in the halls at the Manor. Visitors have left at eight. Most patients are in bed. A few "night wanderers" and "night owls" are tolerated. Aides consider "wanderers" harmless and, besides, "it breaks the monotony." Night owls are alert patients who retire near midnight because "they like to fool around in their rooms." Some watch television. A few play cards.

Bed-and-body work at night involves answering periodic calls for toileting and making bed checks. In making bed checks, aides enter rooms to see "if everything's all right." They are quite flippant about this. Some patients claim to be shocked by such nightly intrusions; others ignore them altogether.

When aides do bed-and-body work, they act rushed and claim to have little time to "fool around" with patients. Indeed, on every shift, the time that floor staff allocates to most bed-and-body work means that *much* must be completed quickly. However, there are also times on every work shift when comparatively little bed-and-body work is done. On days, it's from about 1 to 3 P.M. On P.M.s, it's from 3:30 to 5 and from 9 to 11. On nights, it's from 11:30 P.M. to 4:30 A.M. Floor staff does not carry bed-and-body work over into these hours.

The meaning of being rushed is not linked to the absolute time that floor personnel have available to do their work. Rather, it hinges on the time they allocate to bed-and-body work. Time not spent on such work may be used to answer a few buzzers, but mostly it is used to chat and share each other's company. It is exceptional for floor personnel to spend much time with patients.

When top staff directives or clientele behavior infringe on how floor staff allocates its time, it routinizes the "annoyances."

ROUTINIZING ANNOYANCES

What floor staff considers normal work with clientele differs from floor to floor at the Manor. For example, on the first floor, aides believe that treating all residents' privacy cautiously is normal routine. On the third and fourth floors, this is normal only to the extent that patients are considered alert. Clientele behavior not believed to be a part of normal work routine is treated as an annoyance. Floor staff works to routinize annoyances.

Two types of events lie outside normal routine. One is related to aspects of top staff work or policy that affect the floors. The other are clientele or clientele-related "excesses."

Administrative Annoyances

Top staff periodically issues directives changing or enforcing some existing work policy. They may be related to the direct care of patients, or they may involve the personal behavior of nurses and aides. Directives take the form of memos.

When a directive is issued, copies are usually posted at the back of each nurses' station and somewhere near the employee time clock in the basement. Typically, one of the top staff nurses distributes it. The charge nurse may be informed of or read the memo's content in the process. When a particular charge nurse is notified of a memo placed at the station and she chooses to inform her staff of its contents, it is commonly those aides who happen to be present at the station at the moment who are notified. This may mean only one or two people. She rarely informs everyone on the floor systematically.

The back of the nurses' station often is cluttered with other memos, lists of various sorts (emergency numbers, names of patients' and residents' physicians, bath schedules, names of patients in isolation, beauty shop appointments), and aides' patient and resident loads for the day. Aides are not in the habit of looking for memos there. Rather, in the process of doing bed-and-body work, they consult what they *need* to complete the task in the "normal" fashion to which they are accustomed.

Aides know that top staff places memos at the nurses' station. They also know that the station usually is cluttered. All floor personnel believe that they are rushed. In their relations with top staff, floor personnel often mention it. Both the clutter and the rush serve as excuses by which aides account for not having followed top staff directives, when they have to account for not following them. Since floor staff has no use for directives that alter normal work routine, they mostly ignore them, knowing that they can easily plead ignorance should they ever be made accountable, which does not happen frequently.

Floor personnel are aware of certain rules of patient care that top staff expects them to follow without exception. For example, aides know that, officially, clientele are permitted to smoke only in certain designated areas such as the dining room and some lounges. Also, clientele are supposed to eat either in their rooms or in the dining area, not in hallways or at the nurses' station. When these rules interfere with normal floor routine, aides often break them.

Rule-breaking is conceived by the floor staff to be a practical and circumstantial procedure by which to resolve care dilemmas. It knows it is breaking rules but usually feels the act is "for the good of all concerned."

Take Mary Clark, for example, the twenty-seven-year-old terminal diabetic mentioned in the preceeding chapter. When Mary entered the Manor, she was granted privileges not commonly given to other patients, partly because she is young and partly because she is officially diagnosed as terminal and knows it. She was allowed to eat anything she desired as well as to smoke in her room.

Some time after her initial entry to the home, top staff informed the charge nurse on the floor that Mary was now to be treated like other patients. This meant that she was to smoke only in the dining room. The charge nurse on the floor informed some of the aides of the new directive.

The directive did not dramatically change the aides' routine treatment of the patient. Allowing Mary to smoke in her room had coincided well with normal work routine. Taking her to the dining room to smoke would have meant that one aide's bed-and-body work would have gone unattended. Not only would an aide have had to go through the slow, agonizing process of taking a patient in constant pain to the dining room, she would also have had to sit with her until she finished her cigarette. As one aide stated, "It's just too much trouble when you're rushed all the time." When the new directive was issued, aides saw no reason why a practice that had worked so well before should be discontinued now.

In continuing Mary's old smoking routine, aides took advantage of three conditions. First, top staff (especially the administrator, who issued the new directive) is rarely on the floor. Second, Mary's room is adjacent to the nurses' station, where "we can keep an eye on her anyway." And, third, a few aides mentioned that they would plead ignorance of the new directive if necessary. Floor staff usually does not break rules unless it feels that it has a justification that top staff will accept should they find out about it.

Top staff expects floor staff to chart clientele systematically and occasionally to complete other kinds of records, in addition to doing bed-and-body work. Charting is fairly well routinized on the floors. Its annoyance is reduced by standard entries and casual completion. At the ends of their shifts, aides gather all the charts of clientele assigned to them that day. Charting is treated so perfunctorily that on one occasion a patient who had left the Manor for a week to be treated in a local hospital was charted while he was away. The entries made in his absence read "normal routine," "cares given," and so on.

Other records, however, are grumbled over. The need to complete them is sufficiently irregular to make them annoying as far as the normal work routine on the floor is concerned.

Whenever a patient or resident has an accident such as falling or fainting, an incident report is written. One of the floor nurses may be asked to complete the report if she is considered to be well acquainted with the person involved and the circumstances under which the accident occurred. The report contains a variety of questions. In addition to name and room number, the person filling out the report is asked for the location of the incident, an account of any property involved, the names of witnesses, a description of the incident, and the patient's or resident's condition before it occurred.

For some floor nurses, this last question is especially annoying. Although the item provides five alternative answers—normal, senile, disoriented, sedated, and other—deciding upon the appropriate one is not a simple matter. Members of the floor staff do not routinely think in such general alternatives. Certainly, they talk the language, but its use is situationally determined and is linked to whether work routines are disrupted, not to the alleged absolute psychological state of the individual patient or resident.

On one occasion, Sally Martin (an LPN) is filling out an incident report on Claude Perlo, a patient who had fallen in the hallway that morning. When she comes to the section on the condition of the patient before the incident, she mutters to herself about not knowing "what the hell to put down" and complains that she doesn't "know why I have to fill this out." She looks up from what she's doing and sees Barbara Kemp (an aide) passing in front of the nurses' station, pushing Claude ahead of her. Sally asks Barbara, "Would you say that Claude is senile, disoriented, or normal?" Barbara pushes and shrugs her shoulders, then, after a moment of thought, "I don't know. I'm not sure." Sally is becoming impatient, for she wants to "finish this damn thing so that I can get on with my work." Sally asks Barbara, who is now walking down the hall, "Would you say 'disoriented'?" Barbara shouts back, without even turning her face toward Sally, "Yeah. I guess so." Sally immediately checks that alternative and moves on to quickly finish the rest of the report.

On another occasion, an RN on the third floor fills out an incident report on a patient who fell while trying to crawl over the foot of her bed on the way to the toilet. She asks me what I think she should put down for the patient's behavior before the incident. I answer that I don't really know. A moment passes. Finally, she says, "Well. I'll mark 'normal.' I'm in a hurry and can't spend all day on this kind of stuff."

Top staff usually places the result of PCCs in specific patients' or residents' charts. If their alleged behavior is considered a problem, it is described as either disoriented, confused, or agitated. Behavioral diagnoses include such directives as "use a positive approach" and "give plenty of TLC." Top staff believes these terms and phrases to have meanings independent of the behavior of particular patients. Floor staff, on the other hand, has little or no use for such general connotations. When asked what these terms mean, floor nurses and aides provide definitions that relate to work routines. This is typified by the following.

I am sitting at the nurses' station on the first floor thumbing through a resident's chart. The charge nurse is seated next to me, writing. At one point, I look at the cardex to check what is written there against similar entries on a chart. The behavioral approach on the care plan reads: "Use a positive approach." I asked the nurse, "What does it mean when it says, 'Use a positive approach'?" She hesitates before she answers. Then she says, "I don't know what it means. Who is that you're looking at?" I told her. The nurse explains, "Oh, on her, I guess it means to be firm."

Answers to questions about the meaning of top staff chart and cardex entries on specific patients and residents are as varied as the floor experiences of nurses and aides. Moreover, these experiences shift from day to day. What a positive approach means to one aide is no guarantee that it will mean the same thing to another. The same aide also interprets it differently depending on day-to-day changes in the amount of "trouble" she is having with particular patients or residents.

When a new patient or resident is admitted to the Manor, his entry papers precede him to the floor. The charge nurse is given his admission form, physician's notes, and any hospital records released to the home. Top staff believes that these papers provide a reasonable preview of the client, presumably giving floor personnel an idea of the kind of patient or resident they are going to have to deal with. For the most part, however, floor nurses routinely ignore preentry papers. They find that in practice such information is of little relevance. To them, relevance is linked to normal floor routine.

When new patients or residents are to be admitted to a floor, nurses and aides may grumble about it. It means a disruption of normal work routine until they are settled into their rooms and learn "how to get along on the floor." One time, as I sympathized with their complaints, I happened to be thumbing through a patient's preentry papers at the nurses' station. I cited the physician's diagnosis, which read "CBS," to the personnel and asked what it meant. Claiming to be exasperated with everything that morning, the charge nurse turned to me and said,

> It doesn't mean anything! They put chronic brain syndrome [CBS], CVA [cerebral vascular accident], or ASHD [arteriosclerotic heart disease] on the charts as a diagnosis. Well, thanks a lot! That tells me nothing. So you know that ateriosclerotic disease cuts the blood flow from the brain and that it'll affect their behavior in some way. But that's too general. I still don't know how a pa-

tient will act till they get here and I see them in action myself.

On those occasions when top staff is on the floors, it may make "quick checks" of bed-and-body work. Floor personnel consider this to be annoying because, as they say, "you have to keep on your toes for all kinds of things while they're here." This hampers what floor staff considers to be normal work routine. Usually, floor staff comes off fairly well when such "quick checks" are made. After all, normal routine is chiefly a matter of bed-and-body work and it is "things like that that they are out to spot."

In the event that something is "spotted," floor staff is ready. Unclean rooms, odors, dirty linens on the floors, crusty bedpans, and the like are rarely claimed by aides as their own sloppy work. Blame is routinely put in one of three places. The previous shift may be accused of not doing its work properly. Sometimes, aides who are temporarily employed at the home from the local medical pool are said to be unfamiliar with the particular routines of the Manor. And at other times, aides say that they are so rushed because of their heavy patient loads that "no one could possibly do everything in the time we have."

Clientele Annoyances

Clientele "excesses" are the second type of interference with normal floor routine. Like those that stem from top staff, clientele annoyances are routinized. Floor nurses and aides seek to make whatever patients and residents do a part of bed-and-body work or to isolate it from this work.

Patients who often interfere with floor staff's bed-and-body work are considered agitated and are sedated. To become agitated means to "deliberately" and directly disrupt or unduly lengthen the time considered necessary to do bed-and-body work. It does not refer to patient activity per se. Patients who are as active as agitated ones but who respect the bounds of normal routine on the floors are not sedated.

Some patients at the Manor are considered to have a history of agitation. As a floor nurse said, "No matter what day it is, you just know that they're going to get into something or other, which just makes it hard on everyone." Soon after they are awakened in

the morning, a nurse usually sedates them. Thorazine and Mel-
laril, both tranquilizers, are well known to all floor personnel.

Early in the day shift, it is not unusual for various aides on the
floor to pass the nurses' station and ask, "Did Max get his shot
today?" or "I hope you remembered to give Emma her Thorazine.
I have a lot of work to do, you know." When the nurses forget to
sedate such patients, concerned aides repeatedly remind them of
it early in their shifts. Nurses usually oblige them if they claim to
be busy, "just to get her [an aide] off my back so we can all get
our work done." When they do not, aides may threaten to do
nothing until their request is granted. Floor nurses are quite
sensitive to such threats, since they are likely to be held responsible for "sloppy care" on the floor should it be noticed during quick
rounds by the top staff. As one floor nurse stated to several aides
just before leaving for her break, "Well, I guess I can take my
break now. Everyone's sedated. It'll be quiet for a while." She
looked from one aide to another. No one objected. All were satisfied that the floor was sedated adequately. The nurse then left.

Aides are most concerned about the sedation of agitated patients on days when they are to spend what they believe is a fair
amount of time with them. On those days when agitated patients
are to be bathed, aides consider it imperative that they be sedated. They are less concerned about this on other days.

One morning, a so-called agitated patient who was still dozing
in bed was a source of concern to an aide who was to bathe him.
Soon after she learned of her assignment and the bath schedule,
she approached one of the floor nurses and asked, "Will you give
Mike his Thorazine now so he'll be calm before I give him his
shower. He's kinda agitated this morning. You know how he gives
you that look sometimes. You just know he's going to act up. He's
in bed right now." The nurse walked into Mike's room and gave
him his shot—quick and easy. The aide was obviously relieved.
She thanked the nurse and went about her work.

Patients and residents do not necessarily enter the Manor with
physician's orders for tranquilizers. However, when aides define
them as "troublemakers," they get tranquilizers shortly after.
Tranquilizers are mostly prescribed "PRN," which means that
they may be administered as needed at the discretion of the floor
nurses. In practice, however, the discretion involved is that of the
aide, who asks for, or reminds a floor nurse of "her need" for, a

sedative. From start to finish, the prescription and administration of tranquilizers is controlled indirectly by aides.

Physicians, who are largely ignorant of their patients' daily lives in the home, honor what usually sounds like a reasonable request for medication. When a floor nurse orders a tranquilizer, she explains that the patient or resident "needs it because he's agitated." She never suggests that it's desired because bed-and-body work is at stake. Also, physicians are not as therapeutically oriented to geriatric nursing home patients as they are to younger ones. This makes it relatively easy to obtain "custodial" orders from them.

Floor staff is wary of patients who occasionally "wander off." Wandering off means walking to some place inside or outside the Manor that is not considered one of the usual and acceptable locations where the individual may be found at a moment's notice. To floor staff, each patient has his "usual" places at the Manor. In doing bed-and-body work, nurses and aides depend on them "staying put" there. A nurse on the third floor explained it this way:

> Pardon my French, but where the fuck do you think we'd be if they [patients] didn't have their favorite spots. When we're looking for them, we're right about 100 percent of the time. I'm sure glad it's like that. Can you imagine what it would be like if patients wouldn't stay put in certain places?

The problem that wandering off poses for floor staff is that rectifying it disrupts normal work routine. It takes time to search the floor for a lost patient. Each room must be systematically checked, and if the person is not found on the floor, the entire Manor is searched, floor by floor. Aides on different floors may become involved in the "annoyance." When a building search does not produce the missing patient, he is assumed to have "run away" or "escaped." Several staff members engage in searching the area.

Patients who wander off are not treated the same way as those considered agitated. They don't block bed-and-body work directly. Rather their absence takes aides away from it. The solution to patients who occasionally wander off is to *make* them "stay put."

Aides make patients "stay put" by restraining them. This is done in a variety of ways. Some patients are placed in wheelchairs dressed in a restraining vest that ties to the back of the chair. Some are seated in geriatric chairs that might be likened to "adult highchairs." Some are dressed in restraining vests but tethered to the railing along the hallway or to some other stationary object. Still others are bound, arms and legs, to their beds.

Although all restraints make patients stay put, they do have their drawbacks. For example, restraining patients tends to produce incontinence. Because they are not free to use the toilet themselves, they become dependent on the floor staff for toileting. Staff availability does not always coincide with the need to eliminate. But since cleaning the products of a bowel movement is routine bed-and-body work anyway, it is considered less of an annoyance than searching for patients.

For some patients, being restrained becomes a vicious circle. When they forcefully resist being bound, they are bound further. This, in turn, induces anger and more resistance, which increases floor staff's felt need to make them stay put. In time, such patients are reduced to what floor staff calls "human vegetables."

Floor staff is not unaware of this vicious circle of restraint and resistance. Some even feel quite guilty about what "we have to do to these poor people." The charge nurse on the third floor expressed her sentiments in this way:

> Her family has problems of its own and can't handle the mother. If the family was OK, the mother could have easily lived with them. So, finally, they had to put Ruth in here. She was fine when she first came. She'd walk around and chatted. She had more weight but she's always been a thin lady, though. The family put it in their mother's mind that she should try it for a while. So Ruth always thought that she'd eventually go home. Now that's all she thinks about. At first, when she could walk, she'd go out of doors and elevators and we'd find her wandering around outside. So we had to barricade the doors and restrain her. You know, we're just gradually wasting her away here. And it's no choice of our own. The family can't handle her and they felt so guilty for putting her here that they keep telling her that she can come home eventually. This excites Ruth, who tries to leave the

Manor. So we have to restrain her. The lack of mobility due to restraints is gradually destroying her, and there's not much we can do about it. When we told her doctor about her at first, he said to sedate her. So we sedated her mildly. At the beginning, she was really spirited. She had a cane and when we tried to restrain her, she'd hit us with it and so on. She hit me in the head. We restrained her in her wheelchair and put the brakes on, but she pulls herself along the carpet with her heels. We're just taking the life out of her. Ruth must have been such a spry person but that kind of person just can't be accommodated here. It's the situation. We're guilty and feel guilty and her family is the same. I just don't know what to do. Now the family is taking out their mother's degeneration on us.

When floor staff foresees what it considers to be "trouble for the whole day," it sedates or restrains the potential troublemakers. Not all annoyances are believed to be long term, however. Some are momentary. For example, a patient may be blocking a doorway, or he may not be proceeding through bed-and-body routines at "normal" pace. Floor staff may routinize such momentary annoyances by what it calls "being firm."

Although being firm differs from sedation and restraint in that it is used to routinize momentary, situated annoyances, it is similar to them in another respect. All three routinize annoyances by objectifying the patient. Rather than talking *with* him about the annoyance he is considered to be, floor staff talks *at* him. And in the process, the patient is manipulated physically. He is treated like an object. Floor staff's attitude toward him is similar to what it is toward, for example, a stuck door or a jammed siderail on a bed.

Floor staff's attitude is that, at that moment and in that place, the patient has no significant interests of his own. The only thing considered relevant is the work routine. Floor staff largely ignores the content of what the patient says, although he or she may be spoken *for* in the same way that the Manor's social worker spoke for a patient's "real intentions" to go to a birthday party in an earlier chapter. In speaking *to* the patient, floor staff is highly patronizing and curt, talking down to him or her in short, explosive phrases.

Patients are physically manipulated in various ways. They may be shoved aside. If they are in wheelchairs, they may simply be wheeled to one corner of a room. They may be lifted bodily and placed somewhere. Occasionally, manipulation is symbolic in the sense that it involves an obvious gesture that threatens physical consequences if the patient concerned does not desist from making trouble.

Take the following very common occurrences. At the time of morning when aides claim to be very rushed, two of them stand next to the nurses' station talking with a nurse about two of their patients. Another patient in a wheelchair is coming down the hallway toward them. Once there, the patient asks to be taken to recreation on the fifth floor. Although the aides hear this, they ignore it as they continue their conversation with the nurse. The patient waits a moment and asks again, louder than the first time. The aides show some annoyance. One of them turns to the patient and firmly says, "You don't want to go to recreation now, Freda!" Hearing this, the patient repeats several times, "Yes, I do! Yes, I do!" The other aide then turns to her and admonishes, "Now, Freda. You're just being foolish. You go and rest in your room for a while like a good girl." The patient then repeats that she knows perfectly well what she wants and that there's no reason why she should be treated like a child. As she implores them to take her, one of the aides pushes Freda's wheelchair into the dining room. All the while, Freda is protesting. When they reach the far corner of the room, the aide applies the wheelchair's brakes. She quickly returns to the station and says, "That should keep her out of the way for a minute or two while we disappear down the hall."

On another occasion, several patients are being taken outdoors to "get some air" on a warm, sunny day. The last patient falls behind slightly as the others proceed outside. She hesitates by the doorway, reluctant to leave the building. An aide notices this and returns to the entrance. She tells the patient, "Come on, Anna." Anna does not move but looks apprehensive. The aide calls to her again while slapping her thigh in the manner that dogs are summoned. When Anna still does not budge, the aide becomes furious. She stamps her foot, clenches her fists with gestures of intent to assault, and shouts hatefully, "Anna! You get out here this very minute or else!" Anna proceeds slowly.

Every week at the Manor, there are events that groups of patients and residents from various floors may attend. These include birthday parties on the fifth floor, religious services on the second, visits from the podiatrist on the second, and physical therapy on the fourth. Such events mean that aides must get a number of patients ready and presentable fairly quickly. It also necessitates taking them to their destination, which is often on another floor. Aides consider these building events to be, as they say, "a big pain in the ass."

Annoyances of this type are routinized by herding patients. This occurs in three stages. First, when the time "to go upstairs" (or downstairs) approaches, aides go quickly down the hallways and shout into each relevant room that it's time for whatever event is soon to occur: "Birthday party time! Get ready!" "Time for church! Let's get going now!" After the event has been announced, patients are, as aides typically say, "rounded up." This is the second stage of herding. Each patient is either wheeled or encouraged to walk to the elevator. Sooner or later, a crowd gathers there, waiting and chatting as the rest are rounded up. When this is completed, the third stage begins. Several aides start to move the group en masse. They are packed into the elevator, wheelchair to wheelchair, and taken to the relevant floor. Two or three trips may be necessary before the job is finished.

Herding patients is a form of collective firmness. Little protest is tolerated. When anyone is unduly slow or uncooperative, he is shoved or pulled along. To aides, the important thing is to get them all there as quickly as possible and with the least trouble.

Momentary annoyances are sometimes routinized by bribing troublemakers. Floor staff bribes those who are believed likely to make more trouble if shoved around. Other patients, with whom floor staff is usually firm, are bribed in the process of being physically manipulated. The latter is an alternative to shoving, which is not done for fear of increasing patient ire.

Bribing generally occurs when floor staff knows what troublemakers value highly. For example, in working with patients from day to day on the floors, nurses and aides become aware that one may be quite fond of smoking or having a couple shots of liquor daily, another of going outdoors, and still another of being taken to recreation. For many patients, these are aide-dependent activities. Cigarettes and matches are locked in a drawer behind the nurses' station. The liquor cabinet is in one of the med rooms, which also is locked. Officially, patients are supposed to ask permission to leave the floor, and many need someone's help to do so. Each of these highly valued but aide-dependent things may be used as bribes to contain trouble-making.

Take Kitty Hayes, a third-floor patient who is known to "smoke like a fiend." Several times a day, she approaches the nurses' station and asks whomever is there for two cigarettes. Sometimes she is teased before she is granted her request. Sometimes she is ignored momentarily, because "everyone knows she'll ask again anyway, so you can't possibly forget it." When Kitty is not given cigarettes immediately, she becomes visibly shaken. Her apprehension makes her "shake because she needs a nicotine fix." Kitty is no one's favorite patient.

One afternoon, Kitty wants to telephone her brother about some matter that she considers urgent. She has no money, so she asks the charge nurse at the nurses' station if she can use the nurse's phone to make an urgent outside call. The nurse replies that only the pay phone is for patient use. When Kitty tells her that she has no money for the pay phone, the nurse says, "I'm sorry, but policy is policy. You'll just have to wait until your brother comes to visit you."

Kitty is irate. She leaves the station and walks back to her room, but about fifteen minutes later, she returns. Another nurse is now seated at the station. Kitty explains her problem and asks for permission to use the nurse's phone. Again she is refused. Kitty immediately begins to scream frantically. She walks to the elevator, pushes the button, and shouts that she is leaving "this godforsaken place." Although the nurses and aides present are visibly annoyed at the screaming, none takes her threat too seriously.

When the elevator doors open, Kitty enters and proceeds to leave. Two aides then bolt to the elevator and hold the doors apart. A nurse commands her to return to the hallway. Kitty refuses and begins a high-pitched tirade about her confinement at the Manor: "You're not going to make a goddamn prisoner out of me! Not me, you aren't! If I want to get out of here, I'm going! Let go of those doors, goddamn it!" One of the aides then asks Kitty if she wants a cigarette. Kitty quivers slightly when she hears this. She turns to the aide and says, "Yes, I do. You know I do." The aide then explains, "Well, you better come on out of there, then." Kitty walks to the dining room for her smoke. She's quiet.

Adele Lubinski also was bribed as she was in the process of leaving the floor. Adele is a fourth-floor patient who once was a resident. After she fell and hurt her shoulder, she was transferred to the fourth floor allegedly because staff felt that she needed greater nursing care than could be provided on the first floor. Staff also thought she complained too much to be with other residents.

One morning, Adele decides to remain in bed quite late. This runs into bed-making time. An aide enters her room and curtly says, "Are you going to get up so that we can make the bed?" After a few groan-filled comments, Adele answers, "Here, I'll get up. Oh, I'm so tired." The ward clerk enters the room and glibly compliments Adele, "My! You look spry this morning." Adele turns to the clerk with an irritatingly puzzled look on her face, "What's the matter with you? Of course, I'm OK. Are *you* all right yourself?"

As Adele trudges down the hall toward the nurses' station, she mutters about "all those crazy nurses around here who talk to you like they got no marbles in their heads." At the station, the following exchange takes place with the charge nurse:

Fed up with life on the fourth floor, Adele initially whines that she wants to go home (first floor).

ADELE: I wanna go down on the first floor. I wanna go home. There's nothing wrong with me. I wanna go downstairs. Just because I bumped my shoulder. Sure, I bumped my shoulder but that'll be better. I want my people. I wanna go right now—back over there. I wanna go now. I got my little dress on. [The charge nurse and an aide snicker.] Well, what's wrong with you people? I only have that little black and white dress. Where's the other folks on the first floor? I feel all right now.

NURSE: You're out of breath now.

ADELE: Oh, I've had that for years. I don't wanna make this my home. I wanna go home to my folks. [The maintenance man walks by.] Hey! Man! Why don't you do something! Just because I bumped my shoulder.

NURSE: [Trying to divert Adele's attention] Look at how short of breath you are, Adele.

Adele grows more "short of breath" as she becomes increasingly angry at what she knows are diversion tactics.

ADELE: Oh, I'm always that way when I talk loud! I'm OK!

NURSE: You can't go down there like this. You have to get dressed first.

ADELE: Oh, I'm OK. What's wrong with this?

NURSE: There, there, honey. Why don't we get you all dressed up?

ADELE: Don't give me that honey stuff! I wanna go and see my people!

NURSE: [With sweet indulgence] Well, let's get ready first. OK?

Adele walks back to her room. Soon the whole matter is forgotten.

Some troublemaking is not considered sufficiently annoying by the floor staff to warrant doing much about it. This kind of trouble does not so much directly disrupt bed-and-body work as it does offer a minor irritation to floor staff's personal sensibilities. For the most part, such annoyances are "gotten used to" and finally ignored. They include persistent pulling of call buzzers by certain patients, continual weeping, daily floor pacing, walking around repeating specific words or phrases, and constant complaining.

Take the example of Marlene Barrett. Anyone who spends a few hours on the third floor of the Manor soon learns that Marlene will verbally accost him repeatedly. Typically, as one passes her, she quickly and frantically repeats, "Where's my room? What shall I do? Where shall I go? Where's my room? Where's my room?" Veteran staff members simply say, "3–2–0, 3–2–0," and walk on. This is Marlene's room number. For them, repeating it is "just a matter of habit." Marlene then repeats the number herself for a while until she accosts someone else who passes by.

When floor staff members first encounter Marlene's repetition of her room number, or if they return to the third floor after working on another for some time, they become annoyed with it. Some grow quite impatient and yell, "Just shut up, will you!" or "Go to your room and be quiet!" Eventually, they learn to ignore it altogether. As a third-floor nurse stated: "Barrett goes around all day saying, '3–2–0, 3–2–0.' At first, I heard it so much that I started to hear it in my sleep. After a while, you hear it so much that you don't hear it at all."

Each floor of the Manor, especially three and four, has a certain din that stems from crying, moaning, buzzing, repeated chains of verbiage, and the like. It eventually grows to be part of the unnoticed background of everyday routine.

CONCLUSION

Floor staff, more than top staff or clientele, experience the social complexities that arise when place is not well insulated. As members of the floor staff enter and depart certain places as part of their work, they tacitly raise doubt about whether those places are private or public. Some places, for example, may be considered the private domain of a resident or patient, or believed to be public to certain clientele by those gathered there at the moment. This makes "troubles" for floor staff.

Floor staff conciliates both top staff and clientele in order to guard what it considers normal work routine. This is a highly precarious working policy. It makes no one completely happy, although, in effect, it "puts off" the always present possibility of a breakdown in routine daily life. Floor staff is well aware of the fact that an unharried existence of its own depends on routinizing annoyances from top staff and clientele. This contributes in no small way to the wily attitude of its members.

CHAPTER 5 | Passing Time

In the wide-awake world of daily living at the Manor, each group—top staff, floor personnel, and clientele—has its business to carry on. In their dealing with each other, each group understands and manipulates the affairs of the other groups in terms of its own business. Thus, when top staff deals with floor nurses and aides, the official business at hand is patient care. When floor nurses and aides deal with their superiors, what stands first in their minds is bed-and-body work. And when clientele deal with floor staff, it is their desire to live as proper human beings despite the constraints of institutional living at the Manor that is at stake.

This chapter is concerned with clientele business. Like most people's affairs, that business is carried on in various places. Sometimes clientele do things among themselves, without staff being present. Sometimes they pass time in places where staff officially presides. In either case, what is done is as rational as its context. To understand how reasonable much of everyday living is, even what seems at first glance, to be "crazy," the context or place in which it occurs must be taken into account.

SITTING AROUND

When clientele business does not involve dealing with staff members, clientele typically say that they "sit around." This is not simply a matter of *just* doing nothing. It is much more than that in two ways. First, it constitutes much of the daily living that patients and residents do at the Manor. When they are not in therapy or engaged in ceremonials such as parties, outings, and saying the rosary or at the receiving end of bed-and-body work, they mostly sit around. In terms of clock time, not sitting around may include the 15 to 40 minutes that some clientele spend in therapy of various sorts, the time it takes to complete such bed-and-body work as eating, voiding, or bathing, and the typical hour-long duration of ceremonials. As a third-floor patient put it, "No. It's not easy to lose 'track' of time here. It's just a world of time."

Second, sitting around is more than doing nothing in that its content is varied. Although patients and residents may refer to their lives at the Manor as "sitting," they ordinarily do not *just* sit. Sitting around means such things as talking, dozing, reading, doing what they call "hand work" (crocheting, knitting, sewing), watching, walking, and puttering. Patients and residents take such things quite seriously. Indeed, when sitting around is reduced to what might be described as *just* sitting, without such activities, clientele typically say that "you get kinda nervous for not even having the darnedest little thing to do."

Getting nervous about *just* sitting has commonly known symptoms. First, when patients and residents feel nervous about *just* sitting, they typically whine or groan that they wish they had something to do. Second, they are anything but calm. Some wring their hands. Some walk about aimlessly, as a few put it, "with your head chopped off." Third, persons who claim to be nervous about *just* sitting often try doing something to fill their felt void.

Filling the void that makes persons say they're nervous takes different forms. Some search for usually sympathetic patients or residents and talk or walk with them; some try puttering; others seek the aid of floor staff.

It is the last group who "makes trouble." They approach nurses and aides anxiously, eager to fill their time with anything. They may ask for something that, as one patient put it, "you really don't need, just to see a face and chat a bit." This might mean calling an aide for things such as "unnecessary" toileting, which produces no urine or stool, or "help" in climbing into bed when everyone concerned knows that it can be accomplished without aid. Some clientele follow aides about or loiter at the nurses' station, either conversing or watching or both in order to calm themselves down. Clientele who anxiously "make trouble" for the floor staff in order to avoid *just* sitting are usually described by nurses and aides as "agitated today." Those who often feel nervous about *just* sitting become known as the "agitated patients."

Whether or not "unnecessary" calls for toileting and the like are in fact unnecessary depends on the context in which they are considered. From floor staff's point of view, when a buzzer is answered, the patient involved "better damn well have to void." When he produces only a little waste (such as "only a trickle") or none at all, he is considered to have bothered staff needlessly. Floor staff tends to be impatient with such persons. If they persist in making what staff believes to be unnecessary calls, their buzzers are eventually ignored altogether. Thus begins the process of becoming known as a "nag."

From the patient's point of view, there are two sides to making "unnecessary" calls to floor staff in order to avoid *just* sitting. First, patients do feel that the calls are needed, in the sense that they produce someone who might help them pass the time for a while. But, second, they are often aware too that such calls may be considered unjustifiable to aides who answer them. Patients know why they make such "unnecessary" calls, but when they are asked, "Then what did you buzz for?" they usually don't admit it. Typically, they answer that they thought they "had to go" but that "it just won't come now." In the long run, such accounts are not accepted by aides who are oriented to visible evidence in such matters.

Sitting around is not a chain of unbroken "activity." It is structured about meals. Whether patients and residents say they talk, putter, or doze when they sit around, all they do occurs in reference to mealtimes. Meals are served at approximately 8 A.M., 12 noon, and about 5:30 P.M. Even though trays are often late, all patients and residents know that gathering and eating will occur near those hours. These are three of the most guaranteed events in their daily lives at the Manor. They look forward to them, some with simple pleasure and others with the firm knowledge that "it's something to do here and you can depend on it."

The Daily Cycle

Patients and residents divide their day into three parts, which fall around meals. The first part, morning, is considered the busiest in the sense that sitting around involves a variety of "little things you should do." What clientele mean by "little things" is puttering that seems more worklike than leisurely. Specifically, it includes washing small items of clothing like underwear and handkerchiefs; dressing for the day; paying bills; tidying up one's room; and catching up on the news. For many patients and residents, such tasks are likely to fill a good part of the morning. Each is done slowly and methodically.

About eleven o'clock, residents begin thinking about lunch. For some, the next hour is taken up with either preparing to go to the dining room or simply waiting around for the sound of trays coming up the elevator to the dining room. Patients, on the other hand, are reminded by aides that noon is approaching. When they are told this, those that are able to begin to walk slowly down the hallway to the dining room. For many, this is a tedious task. It is about 130 feet from one end of the hallway to the dining room. Once patients reach the dining room, they begin a fairly long period of sitting and waiting for trays.

The second part of the day, afternoon, is considered the longest. Afternoons are said to "just drag by." Sitting around at this time more closely approximates *just* sitting than it does in the morning or evening. In the morning, clientele look forward to and prepare themselves for the day. This "goal in mind" helps to pass time. By the afternoon, however, those who are capable of it have already completed all "those little things that you should do." All that remains on an ordinary day-to-day basis is to think about supper. And, as they say, "That's such a long way off." For most, passing time in the afternoon is a matter of killing five or six hours.

Evening is the third part of the day. This is the time from supper to bed. For most, it ranges from one to four hours. Some patients and residents begin to retire at 7 P.M. By about 10 o'clock, most are sleeping. Those patients who are put to bed by aides are usually retired shortly after eight o'clock, when visiting hours end. As one aide put it, "When the families leave, you put grandma and grandpa to bed and by about 9 o'clock, things are all kinda quiet." Evening is not usually felt to drag by. It is taken up with a variety of activities: visiting, chatting, playing cards, and getting ready for bed.

Altogether, a fair amount of the time in which sitting around is done is spent in preparation at the Manor. This occurs in the mornings and evenings. In the morning, clientele prepare for the day. In the evening, they prepare for bed. In between, time drags.

When patients and residents talk about their day, it is evident that they consider any one day to be much the same as any other. All emphasize, and some even are slightly amazed at, how uniform day-to-day life is at the Manor. This uniformity includes the weekends. As they emphasize over and over again, "No matter when you're talking about, each day is the same old routine." To them this means, for the most part, "You eat, sleep, and sit around." The following excerpts from conversations with patients and residents show the flavor of what it means to sit around from meal to meal.

Rachel Wynn [resident]: I get up at six, and I get ready. Then, at seven, I call Daisy [roommate]. Then, she gets ready. That's why I don't have to speed. I've had to slow up. And then we have breakfast. After that, we come back in here [their room]. See, the mornings go quickly. The afternoons seem to drag. I don't do any fancy work [knitting, crocheting, etc.]. Having worked, you know, and then my parents weren't too well, and then when I'd come home there were always little things to do. I used to read a good deal more than I do now and do crossword puzzles. I kind of got away from that a little bit. After breakfast, we come back in here and I straighten around . . . maybe dust a little better and do things. Nothing very much. That's what's hard. We go for a walk mostly every morning. I go with Mrs. Doherty because I can't walk alone. The doctor didn't want me to go out alone. Daisy can't walk as far as I can, and so sometimes we go just a little ways and she comes along. Then after lunch, let's see. What do we do? Sometimes we read a little bit. Or else if it's nice, we go out and sit out, and . . . the afternoons are long. They drag. In the evening, we usually play cards or something. We did later on in the afternoon—maybe from four until dinner time, we'd play cards. Well, you see, you have your lunch and then it's from one till six o'clock. You can't keep busy all that time. In the morning, you can straighten a drawer, or putter around, or find something to do. But the afternoons drag, really drag, and we aren't able to walk that far or walk that long, you know. If you've taken a walk in the morning for about half an hour or so, you're tired. Close to six o'clock, we have dinner. Then, in the evening, we read the paper and usually play cards or something. I've been playing bridge with Lenore down the hall and Margaret Daley and them. Last night, someone couldn't come. So they asked me. We never play later than nine o'clock. A little after nine, of course, I like to go to bed—a little earlier than she [Daisy] does. Lately, we watch programs. We've been listening to the main program that's been on [Watergate testimony]. We've enjoyed it too—I mean the testimony and that. So we get to bed closer to ten than nine.

Belle Kelonen [patient]: It's a bit too quiet here. Now, at home, there's the carpet to take care of. There's the dusting on the mahogany stuff. I got all mahogany. And there's my room to take care of. My sister takes care of her own room. Well, here, I tried to fix my bed one morning and the girl [aide] says, "Oh, you better let me do it." So I quit. Let 'em do it if they wanna do it. But they sure keep their carpets nice here. They vacuum everyday. Oh here, I do practically nothing. I'd rather do a little something. But I wipe off the stuff that I think looks dusty because doesn't the air condition throw a little dust? Now what do I do in the afternoon? That's a big question. What should I do? There's nothing to do. So I take myself a nap and think over this big mistake that I made. What is there to do here? I had these books here. I sat outside and read some of the movie books. But, outside of that, what? You can't do nothing because I don't think they let ya. So what are you supposed to do? I cover the bed if I upset it. I cover it over again, you know. This is a very nice place. After dinner, I don't do anything. I come in here [her room] and I undress and I lounge around and flop on the bed because it's rest that I need. I'll never put on any weight if I don't rest. So that's what I do. I rest.

Virginia Cramer [patient]: I think it's probably about half past six when I get up. Then I just sit indefinitely. Some days, I don't feel very good. I just wait for breakfast in my room. Well, I suppose it must be special privileges. I don't know. I don't care to eat in the dining room. You get in there and you can't get out. Well, they have certain ones to wheel around and somebody wants something, I suppose. So I just sit and wait till they can get to me. Mrs. Someone . . . well, she didn't come up yesterday from breakfast till after lunch. Well, that must have been an awful long time to sit. Of course, she can't talk. In the afternoon some of the help has to come in [P.M. shift]. And today one of the girls took me for a ride up and down the hall. Then I go to bed after supper about seven. I think I'm in bed by seven.

Barry Hampton [patient]: I got up at 2 o'clock this morning. I don't sleep. I lay in bed. Every little while I look at the clock. Boy, does time go by slow. Fifteen minutes is like four hours. They come around to wake us up around five-thirty or six. I usually get out of bed when they come in for him [roommate] to give him some pills. Of course, I never did sleep much. Breakfast is supposed to be at seven-thirty, but it gets to be 8 o'clock once in a while. We wait all the time. They get us down there at quarter to seven. We wait for breakfast for 45 minutes. After breakfast, we just sit down in front there. We watch the traffic. We sit down and listen to the women talk. They talk. Ah, God! What they talk about! I go to therapy. We go upstairs to the fifth floor. One day it was on the fourth floor. That passes an hour or an hour-and-a-half away. In the afternoon we sit down in front. And then I got company coming. After supper we sit down in the lounge and listen to them quarrel. That's all. We go to bed early—around 8 o'clock.

Gus Marsh [resident]: I eat breakfast. I smoke about twenty cigarettes, or ten anyway. At the front end [lobby] with the others around, we talk. At about half past nine, I come to my room and shave and make my bed. Then it's coffee time. So I take my straw hat and go out the back door. I go to Sam's for coffee. It's close by. Ya watch the people and smoke a couple of cigarettes. After a couple of weeks, ya get to know the waitresses a little. They'll have something to say about the ball game or some general subject. And then I walk around the block and come home and wait for lunch. After lunch ya got all afternoon with nothing to do. I lay down a little. I don't want to sleep if I can help it. I just lay there and relax. Then I come out and smoke. Lately, the weather's nice. They [residents] take their chairs outside. They haven't got no lawn chairs or nothing. They [top staff] say they have them ordered and this and that. My God! It's been open for a while now. They should have lawn chairs delivered by this time of year. They're so slow in getting anything done around here. The administrator don't see things. He's running around with those sheets of paper. Then you don't see him for a day or two. Maybe he's out on some business or something. I have my coffee again at 3 o'clock. I'm a coffee drinker. And then this little girl Dorothy [a resident], she come along with me yesterday. Then we sit there and talk and jabber. Then we come back the other way. And then we just lay around. We got to wait for supper. Ya visit with one a little and that one. What can you do? We sit around and sit around and that's it. Some of them are in their room and watching certain programs. That's what most of them do. They just lay on their bed and watch television. After supper, Johnny [his nephew] comes down and visits. Dorothy had her nephew come down. He's taking care of her affairs. She got money, ya know.

Homer Wilson [resident]: They knock on the door at 7 o'clock. "Mr. Wilson. Seven o'clock. Time to get up and have yourself weighed before breakfast." So you dress and you shave and have yourself ready. You go out and you're weighed. Then you go to breakfast and you have your breakfast. Then you're free to wander around here like a lost sheep, you know, till you get ready to go to bed again, or until noontime when you eat again. They weigh you every morning. I don't know why they do or if they do it to all patients, but I'm weighed every morning. Of course, you see, when you're here you're under doctor's supervision. You can have your own doctor and he lays the plans of what to do and what not to do. Everything is left at the desk [nurses' station]. Any pills you're to take is left at the desk. You want an aspirin tablet, you can have it. If you have a headache and you want it . . . but you can't have it in your room. You gotta go to the desk and get it. So you go there and they very politely give you your aspirin. All the other pills and everything else is by doctor's orders only. So you just lie around. What is there to do? I can't go out and jump rope. You just wait for lunch, I guess. Lunch won't come to me. That's the next step: to eat at noon. Then you go and sit on your ass and wait for the next one. You go from one meal to the next. That's about it. The ladies, they go and probably do a little knitting or sewing, sewing a button, or something. That's their life. But a man, he goes out in the outer lobby and picks up the paper and reads the morning paper if he wishes to, which I usually do. I take my paper and take my paper to my wife's room [third floor] and sit down and read the paper. After lunch, you just lie around some more. There's nothing to do. I haven't any TV. I've lost all interest in TV. I didn't even take my beautiful TV from home. I have a beautiful, large color television. I gave it to my youngest son. Of course, losing your wife [his wife is dying on the third floor], everything goes with it. You get into that funny, sliding corner when you're not interested any more. We were just like this. [Wrings fingers together tightly.] We used to have certain programs we'd listen to. And I've lost all interest in it because she isn't there with me. That's all I can say. For some reason or other, the interest in it is gone. Even like Friday nights, we would never miss Lawrence Welk. Now I can take Friday after Friday and never even miss it because, without her, the interest is gone. We had things in common

like our garden and our home and our grandchildren
. . . like any other married couple would have.

Don Staats [resident]: Oh, ya get up about quarter to
seven, 7 o'clock. Eat breakfast, 8 o'clock, round about,
before or after. Ain't no big rush. Then I wait till noon.
There's nothin' to do. Read the paper. I get the *Courier.*
I don't get the *Daily.* I give the *Courier* to a lady down
here and then she gives me the *Daily* at night when she
gets done with it. That way, I don't have to buy two
papers. So we change one with the other, see. Sunday
I buy my paper. I'm gonna cut that out too. I'm not gonna
pay the *Daily* 40 cents for all them goddamn ads they got
in there. Christ! You open the three front sections that
they got . . . well, they got somethin' written in each
one of them. There's mostly all ads in each one of them
too. So what am I buying the goddamn *Daily* for? To
look at the ads? The rest of the crap that's in there, what
the dickens! I don't wanna buy no home. I don't wanna
sell no automobiles. I can pick up the *Daily* when somebody else gets through with it. Then, I do like always.
Sit here and look. Find something to look at. I spend
a lot of time sittin' outside there with Blondie [woman
friend on the floor]. Look at the automobiles goin' by
and the people. There ain't much people goin' by. They
all got cars. They don't have to walk now. I gotta like it.
I got nothin' else to do. There's some nice lookin' dames
out there. I wouldn't mind having one of them sit along
side of me, or sit on my lap, you know, if there wasn't
anybody lookin'. Then I do the same as always. Look
around. Supper time is six [officially, about five-thirty].
Yeah—eight, twelve, and six. Not always on the dot.
Sometimes about ten after. After supper sometimes
maybe the children come over and spend about a half
hour or so. We sit down in the lobby [lounge] and chat
a little bit or so. They got a television down there and I
got one here too. Well I watch it here sometimes. Sometimes the women'll come in the lounge or a couple of
men we got on the floor. There's only five of us here
[men]—five or six I guess now. Oh, them men talk a

little bit, not much. They're not much of talkers. I go to bed around 10 o'clock. Some of the women here go to bed already at 7 o'clock, 7:30, or 8 o'clock. I said, "You can go to bed for all I care. I ain't goin' to bed yet." When I go to bed, I wanna sleep. I don't wanna lay there and roll around from one side to the other. I'd fall out of the damn thing.

When patients and residents talk about their day, they suggest that it feels most unnatural in the afternoons. This feeling is related to what felt normal for most of them before entering the Manor. As one of them put it,

You know, it's kinda hard to take this life when you're used to being busy most of the day. The only time that you really feel right in a place like this is after supper. It's like before. You know. You sit around and read the evening paper, maybe visit a little.

Getting up at seven and "going to work" in the everyday world of adult life has its affinities with awakening early at the Manor and "doing all the little things you have to" before the day goes on. However, when this is finished, the similarities end. Evenings at the Manor also have affinities with evenings in many American homes after daytime working hours.

There is another side to this. Visitors to the Manor and floor staff occasionally comment on how different the mood of the floors is at different times. Typically, they say that in the afternoons "the feeling you get about life here is a lot different than if you come later in the day." They mention that patients and residents seem to drift aimlessly after noon. Certainly, some appear to do this all the time. But what visitors and staff are referring to is not the relative proportion of drifters and nondrifters from hour to hour; rather, they are talking about atmosphere. As one relative said:

When I visit my mother in the afternoon, you tend to notice things more. Things kinda hit you in the face like all those people just sitting around in wheelchairs or just sitting up front looking outside all day. At night I feel more at home when I come. They might still be sitting around, but then. . . . Oh, I don't know . . . well, you sit around with 'em. It's like a visit.

Keeping Track of Time

Patients and residents often comment on or ask each other and staff members what day it is. Although the comments take a variety of forms, the responses to the naming of a day are likely to be the same. For example, in chatting, one patient asks an aide the day of the week. The aide, being in a teasing mood, says, "What day do you think it is, Lydia?" Lydia answers that she doesn't know. The aide then reports that it's Wednesday. Lydia looks slightly surprised and comments, "Oh, it is? For some reason or other, I thought it was Sunday. I don't know why, though." Or on another occasion, two patients sit in the lounge on the third floor. All is quiet, then one asks the other, "Is this Sunday? It sure feels like it." The other answers, "I know what you mean—just lazying around with nothing to do." The first one responds, "Yeah. You just never know what to do with yourself on days like this." After a pause, the other answers with a sigh, "You said a mouthful there. Aren't they just all the same." Life at the Manor is said to most closely resemble Sunday. This is evident in most casual conversation when the topic arises.

The world of time for patients and residents depends on whether or not they have time-related obligations. Those who maintain outside ties that obligate them to keep track of clock time do so. This is more common among residents than patients, but it is not exclusive to them. When clientele feel that they must be on time in order to successfully accomplish a visit with someone in the clock-oriented, workaday world outside the Manor, such as a dentist, lawyer, or friend, they keep track of it. When one has made appointments it is reasonable to keep them. When one is to have lunch with a friend who has a limited amount of time to spend, it is important to maximize one's presence with her.

A few patients and residents keep track of clock time for reasons related to Manor obligations. For instance, some have television programs that they watch religiously, especially afternoon soap operas. As the time for the programs approaches, they settle themselves to watch: television sets are turned on; positions are taken; "hand work" may be readied to occupy one's fingers during the program. Before a program begins, a fairly elaborate preparation ritual may be performed, with periodic glances at the clock.

For the most part, clientele with no outside obligations and no time-related ones in the Manor do not keep track of clock time. There are rare exceptions. A few know the time and say that they keep track of it despite the absence of time-related obligations "because I enjoy it." To them, keeping track of time is felt to be one of "those little things that you do to fill your day." They wear watches and consult them in the process of looking ahead to such daily events as dining and retiring. They take it upon themselves to correct those in their company who make "errors" in estimating the hour of the day. They may remind others in casual conversation that it's "two hours to supper," or that it's "ten minutes till bingo" on those days of the week when the game is played.

Clientele may have two worlds of time at the Manor. One is clock time. The other is the pace of normal work routine on the floor as set by nurses and aides. Patient and residents who maintain clock-time-related obligations carry on their lives in both. In the first world, they keep track of time themselves. In the other, they depend on floor personnel for pacing. Clientele who do not maintain clock-time-related obligations and do not keep time as "something to do" live only in the world of normal work routine.

The time world of normal work routine is believed by most patients and residents to be as normal as clock time—each in its proper circumstances. When it is considered important, one keeps clock time, but in everyday life on the floors, it is believed to be useless and often a hindrance to "getting along." Two patients put it this way:

> For what time? Oh, I got my watch. Yeah, they [relatives] got me that so I. . . . It's not exactly important to know what time it is. I wouldn't say exactly. Because they [aides] come and get you when your mealtime is ready. They take us and bring us back and then we sit. Yeah. They come and do. We don't have to keep track of time—not for that reason. It's just nice to know. You know . . . just to have time. But, otherwise, they come and get us here. I do say that. I haven't forgotten what day it is. Not so far! [laughs] So far, no. It's important when we know when company is coming, more or less, you know. I've had company. I must say, lots. I do have a lot of com-

pany. But on the weekends it's the most. They come mostly in the evening. Yeah.

I lose track of time. I don't know the date. I don't remember the dates. I have no calendar and I don't remember things. I got my watch here. So I try to wind it and look at it, but sometimes I get confused too. It doesn't matter that much anyway. Downstairs [same floor] in the dining room, or somewheres else, they should have a clock to look at once in a while. They do have one at the desk [nurses' station] there, but I have to wheel myself way over there to find out. And I have a problem with this wheelchair. . . . Oh, that wheelchair was killing me. Everytime I was going somewheres . . . you got to take care of yourself; you need that; you need that exercise. . . . That chair bothered me. I dress myself. I do everything myself. I go to the lavatory. I wipe myself. Only it's hard for me to wheel myself to the closet to get my clothes. So the girls [aides] will get it for me. Many times I forget what day it is. Even this morning I didn't know what day it was. It doesn't make any difference because I don't go out any place. I just remember when my sister's coming. That's the only thing to remember. Now she's coming next week Wednesday. She's gotta take me to the dentist again. And they're real nice. They help her with the wheelchair to take me over to the doctor through the street. Time doesn't matter because I don't go out any place, unless here for bingo and they always take me up there. Then I go to church [second floor]. I just love that church and I'm satisfied. I go to the elevator and they take me. When there's a rosary, they come and let me know if I want to go to rosary. If I wanna go, then they wheel me over. I don't know when they have the rosary so they come and let me know. I remember church. Every Sunday I remember and go there. See now today is Friday—I remember—I don't wanna miss church because I'm a Catholic. And I go to Communion every Sunday. I like that priest. I don't know his name. And I pray to God for my health. [Weeps.]

Two kinds of patients or residents at the Manor do not allow floor staff to pace normal floor routines. One is some newly admitted clientele. They do not leave the world of clock time immediately upon entering the Manor. They tend to want their calls answered and "things done on time" and are considered temporarily "confused" by the staff. Through experience, most learn to leave time on the floors to nurses and aides. In the process, their "confusion" subsides. The other kind is those who "make trouble" because they are obstinate timekeepers; they are annoyances that floor staff learns to routinize. As one floor nurse said, "They refuse to see that we'll get to them in good time."

Eating

As one might expect in any social setting where casual talk occurs, patients' and residents' conversations dwell on the main events of their daily lives. A great deal of casual talk at the Manor centers on dining. This involves judgments of food, before, during, and after meals. As one resident put it,

> There're two favorite topics of conversation in a place like this: food, and aches and pains. Of course, some of them like to talk about other things too. You've got the people that are always talking about their teeth . . . you know, their dentures . . . and some only have their bowels on their minds. It's hard at first to get used to, but then it seems like a normal topic of conversation. All's everyone has to do here is wait for one meal after another. They leave breakfast and tell each other they'll see each other at lunch. They leave lunch and say the same about supper. And the same at supper. The next day it starts over again.

Talk about food occurs in many places in the Manor. It is carried on, in anticipation, in those places where clientele wait for meals, such as their own rooms, the lobby, and the lounges, as well as in the dining room itself. It takes place rather forcefully while meals are being eaten. Talk about food also constitutes a major part of the leisure conversation that clientele make throughout the day between meals.

At the Manor, clientele are not aware of the menu for any meal before they actually see their food on the table. As a result, there is much premeal debate about food while patients and residents sit around waiting for trays. Premeal talk of food has its typical pattern. In a gathering, it commonly begins with someone sarcastically raising the question of what will be served today. The speaker's intonation makes it plain that those gathered take for granted that the food probably will be unsatisfactory. Sometimes the question is hostile in addition to being sarcastic. For example, it is not unusual for someone to initiate premeal food talk with: "I wonder what poison they're going to force down our throats today?" or "Are you ready to choke?"

After the initial question is asked, it is usually repeated a few times or restated by others: "Yeah, what poison?" "They'll probably croak us yet!" "Choke is right." " 'Ready to choke?' You mean, 'Ready to die?' " This sometimes leads to a brief session of what might be described as initial-question-one-upmanship. Each participant tries to reconstruct the initial question in such a way that it is both more sarcastic and more humorous than before. For instance, on one occasion, a resident topped everyone else with, "Here they keep you alive with pills and kill you with the food."

Next, participants relate what they anticipate to past experiences with what they consider bad meals. They remind each other of the well-known occasions when "something really awful" was served. Their recollections of "awful food" are reminiscent of top staff's stories about "crazy" clientele behavior. Anecdotes are told and retold and suggest to the participants in the conversation that they see the world at hand in much the same way.

When food trays are about to be distributed, a relative hush comes over the dining room. At the Manor, entrees are placed on heated plates that have covers. Clientele don't know what the main course is until they either remove the cover themselves or hear the comments of others in the room who already have done so. This is a moment of moans and groans, some of which are contradictory: "Not this again!" "It's about time they served us chicken." "There's just too much on this plate. It ruins my appetite." "They didn't give me any bread." "This meat patty is too dry." "Sawdust again."

Food served at any meal varies somewhat according to the preferences of clientele and the dietary orders from physicians. Although patients and residents often are aware of their own dietary restrictions, they may ignore these restrictions at the table, and instead grumble about what they are served as compared to others. Clientele also share food. When a friend has been "unduly cheated" of something that everyone else has been served, he is offered a portion from another's plate as part of the social obligations felt between friends, regardless of diet.

Time spent in premeal and leisure talk about food contrasts with the amount of time spent eating. Once clientele realize what they are being fed, they proceed to consume the meal rapidly. Consumption is individually paced. Neither among patients nor among residents is there any informal rule that governs how fast or slowly one eats. When a person's tray is placed in front of him, he begins to eat immediately without waiting for anyone else's tray at his table to arrive. Because it may take as long as 15 or 20 minutes to distribute all trays, some persons may be just receiving their food as others at the same table are about to leave. When a person has finished his meal, he may simply rise and depart. Although some make comments on the individualistic pace of eating, no one objects to it. When a tray arrives, everyone expects the person served to begin. When he has finished, he is believed to have every right to simply leave if he wishes.

Residents and ambulatory patients do not all enter and leave the dining room immediately before and after meals are served. On the first floor, some residents begin drifting in and sitting at their tables about a half-hour before mealtime. Some linger afterward to smoke and/or gossip. The majority, however, enter and depart fairly abruptly.

On the third and fourth floors, sitting around in the dining room is more typical. A few ambulatory patients enter the dining room at will several times between meals and *just* sit in their usual chairs, staring aimlessly ahead. They walk back and forth from their own rooms to the dining area most of the day.

Tillie Brook is typical of these patients. After she awakens in the morning and is helped to dress, she walks to her place in the dining room. It may be about 7 A.M. She sits, hands in her lap, and waits silently for breakfast. When her tray arrives, she eats quietly; she continues to sit even after she is finished. After trays are collected and most patients have departed the area, the room becomes fairly quiet. Tillie dozes in her chair. About midmorning, she is likely to walk back to her room, but shortly afterward she returns to her place in the dining room and resumes her silent wait. When noon trays arrive, she has been present in her chair for a long while. Her afternoons and evenings are spent the same way. Occasionally, she paces nervously between her room and the dining area. Along the way, she often stops briefly at the nurses' station and comments haltingly on her unsettled feelings. The nurses acknowledge her sentiments as she moves on.

Some patients pass a fair amount of their day sitting around in the dining room in their wheelchairs, especially those who do not have the strength to wheel themselves easily about or who are otherwise physically disabled. Like Tillie, these patients *just* sit, but they are usually much angrier about it than the ambulatory patients who do so. They also claim to be nervous, but they place the blame for their feelings directly on the floor staff. Ambulatory patients do not; they don't speak of blame but only of passing time.

Each floor of the Manor has one or two patients or residents who pass time in the dining room, during and around meals, doing small tasks. For example, on the first floor, Steve Shore waits by the elevators until he hears the tray carts arrive from the basement. There are usually three of them. He helps the busboy wheel them down to the dining room and then helps to distribute them to the other residents. On the third floor, Sal Zenda makes it his business to collect trays after meals. He is also quite solicitous of patients' requests for such things as missing eating utensils and additional coffee. On the fourth floor, Lulu Mills is the "perfect hostess" at times. When she has finished her own meal, she fetches one of the coffee carafes and cordially pours for any patient who she feels needs more to drink. Lulu proceeds from table to table with her characteristic trudge, humorously teasing as she does her self-appointed job.

Walking

Taking walks passes time for some clientele. Those who take walks give two reasons for it. According to them, walking is beneficial to one's health; it is good exercise. As they often ask, "In a place like this, how else are you going to keep yourself in good shape?" But they also hasten to add that it passes the time.

Patients and residents who take walks do so mostly on a scheduled basis. This means that they set aside a certain part of the day for it. For some, it is done a "little after breakfast." For others, it comes in the afternoon. Little or no walking of any kind is done after supper. The timing of walks, like most clientele activity at the Manor, is contingent on the pace of normal floor routine. When meals come late, for example, walks do too.

Walks occur in two locations. One is outside the Manor, usually either on its grounds or in the near vicinity. The other location is any one of the Manor's hallways. Because of their ambulatory differences, residents more commonly take their walks outdoors, whereas patients do so in hallways on their floors. There are, of course, exceptions, like residents who consider themselves not sufficiently stable on their feet to hazard the outdoors and patients who believe that, except for their official floor location, they are in every way as competent as residents.

Walking out-of-doors is dependent on the weather. When it is too wet or too cold, they are not taken. This doesn't necessarily mean that on these occasions clientele who normally walk outdoors grow "nervous," as they say, because they have to *just* sit. They become "nervous" only when they find nothing else to fill the time usually set aside for taking walks. This is more common on rainy days than in winter. To residents, rain not only prevents outdoor activity, it also provides little of interest to watch from indoors. Winter is another matter, especially during heavy snows, for it means sitting together in the various lounges and lobby and "keeping an eye" on the progress of city snow clearance crews, the Manor's maintenance man, drivers, and pedestrians as they make their way through inclement weather. It means talk and conviviality. Some make "keeping track" of snow clearance progress a self-appointed task as they take it upon themselves to be purveyors of snow news on the floors.

Walking out-of-doors is not commonly done alone. Patients and residents accompany each other. When one of those accustomed to walking with another cannot do so because she is sick, visiting her family, entertaining visitors in her room, and the like, walking is temporarily suspended. Persons who make a habit of taking walks together refer to each other as "walking partners."

Outdoor walks begin when one walking partner says to another at the accustomed time, "Are you ready?" The implication is "to go out for a walk." Despite outside temperatures that may be as high as the nineties, a common precaution that walkers take before they depart is to "put a little something on in case it gets cool or something." This usually means that walks are taken wearing such items of clothing as light coats, sweaters, or kerchiefs. "Putting a little something on" also depends on the distance clientele expect themselves to be "from home," that is, the Manor. If the walkers are staying on the Manor's grounds, they dress more lightly. What is involved in dressing for walks out-of-doors is not just the current state of the weather but also one's relative inability to quickly seek shelter should weather become somewhat inclement.

Women who take walks do so arm-in-arm; men who take walks do not cling to each other. Outdoor walks vary in length. There are a few well-known routes. One is the block. Another is the half-block. The least walked routes are those that take persons to the nearby shopping center or local coffee shop on the next block.

When outdoor walkers return to the Manor, they invariably report to others about either or both of two kinds of events. They cite the length of the walk. If it has been what they believe to be exceptionally long, such as an extra block or "all the way to the shopping center and back," they boast of their achievement. Talk about such long walks may pass much of the day on which they are accomplished. Indeed, the few walks that clientele consider to be extraordinarily lengthy are part of their anecdotal history. Other walks are likely to be compared with them.

Returning outdoor walkers also describe any "unusual happenings" that occurred along the way. Like boastful talk of length, recollections of "unusual happenings" pass time. Take Dorothy Porath and Martha Cush. They regularly walk the block in the early afternoon. On one occasion, at the end of the block away from the home, Martha, who has angina, began having chest pains, and she had to sit down at the curb. Dorothy hovered over her until the pain subsided. When they returned to the building, both talked in detail for hours about the features of the attack, the curb-sitting, what passers-by might have thought, Dorothy's feelings of helplessness, their thoughts during the attack, and their strategy for "getting home."

Indoor walks have a pattern similar to outdoor ones, except that they are more likely to be done alone and postwalk talk mostly dwells on length and not on "unusual happenings." Before the walk is taken, clientele dress appropriately. The hallway is considered to be a public place. Like other public areas such as the street, one does not venture there in one's "house" clothing. During the walk, other clientele and members of the staff along the way are greeted and engaged in brief chats. Typically, the walkers announce that it is their daily walk they're taking. For example, when Eileen Schell walks by the nurses' station as she goes from one end of the hallway to the other, she commonly says to whomever is there, "This is sure a long walk. But I walk this hall four or five times a day. It's the only exercise I get and its good for me. Anyway, it does pass the time nicely, you know." From beginning to end, an indoor walk the entire length of the hallway together with casual talk along the way may pass 20 and sometimes 30 minutes.

Sleeping

Sleeping is another way that patients and residents pass time during the day. Sleeping may occur in one's own bed or another's, in lounges, in the lobby, in hallways, in the dining room, and at the nurses' station. Some of it is regularized and some is sporadic. For example, many residents and patients take a nap after lunch. One the other hand, at any location on the floors, seated clientele are likely to doze off if things become monotonous.

On a day when, as clientele says, "nothing much is happening" (which is quite often) and the rush of bed-and-body work is momentarily over, several patients are likely to be sitting in wheelchairs or dining room chairs in the vicinity of the nurses' station, simply watching passers-by. As time progresses, they typically fall asleep, their heads dropping forward or to one side. Some snore. Some drop items that they were holding before they fell asleep. The scene lasts until floor staff is ready to get on with the next stage of normal work routine.

Occasionally, a patient becomes very tired while walking from one end of the hall to another. Some tire from the slightest exertion. Before reaching his own room, he may decide that he must rest, and if he is near some other patient's room, he may enter and nap in that bed. A few patients habitually sleep or doze at any place on the floor that they find convenient. These may be public places or private rooms.

When patients pass time by sleeping in places considered private by others, quite a commotion may be created. It begins with the discovery of the place violation by its official occupant. The violator is told forcefully to leave immediately, that is, to "get out of my bed!" Often, the one who has been sleeping there awakens alarmed and wonders why he is being shouted at. The two typically become involved in an argument, in part over the rudeness of the awakening and in part over the "gall" shown by the intruder in using someone's private room when "you have a bed of your own!"

If the matter is not soon resolved, floor staff may become involved. This happens in two ways. When the yelling is loud enough to be heard by aides or nurses somewhere else on the floor, they investigate the matter if they are not too busy and then clear the room of its unofficial occupant. When floor staff doesn't hear the commotion and come on its own, the room's occupant rushes to the desk and "reports" the violator, whereupon a nurse or aide may come to rectify the situation. As in other situations, whether floor staff goes to the room depends on how busy its members feel they are. When they consider themselves too busy to "fool around with patients' problems with each other," they dismiss the complainant with such remarks as: "Now, really! She's only taking a little nap." "Velma is harmless. Why don't you just go down the hall for a while. She's only resting for a minute or two." "Is that all the fuss is about? Just calm yourself for a while." In response to such problems, floor staff invokes official or unofficial reasons, depending on its needs at the moment.

The amount of sleeping that patients and residents do to pass time varies considerably. Some nap only in the early afternoon for about an hour. Others return to their made beds, carefully sleep *on* them most of the morning and afternoon, and retire right after their evening meal.

Patients and residents who "sleep their whole day away" are considered by others as "whiling all their time away." They are used as examples of persons who "don't know what to do with themselves." *Just* sleeping all day may pass time, but it lends no prestige to those who do it. Others boast that they "don't sleep around all day like some others in this place do." This is especially true of residents who believe themselves to be more "normal" adults than patients and, consequently, more capable of doing something with their lives than they are.

Where one sleeps to pass time makes a difference in how the sleeping is evaluated by others. Sleeping in bed most of the day day is judged negatively, but spending nearly as much time sleeping in the Manor's lobby or lounges is considered just a matter of dozing off. The former is believed to be a deliberate plan to *just* sleep, whereas the latter is treated as one of those things that "happens" when it gets warm and quiet. Dozing off is defined as an event that "happens," even though for some patients and residents it happens fairly systematically. At certain times throughout the day, they may be found dozing in specific public places at the Manor.

There is another side to the difference between sleeping in one's room and sleeping in public places. When someone is discovered to be sleeping in his own room, he is not disturbed unless time is close for some event such as meals or bingo, which others believe he should attend. When someone is seen sleeping in a public place, he is considered to have just dozed off and thus to be available for awakening at any time. Presence in a public place signifies that one is open to visiting and only momentarily (sometimes for over an hour) inattentive to personal exchange.

Watching

Patients and residents also pass time by what they call watching or looking. The practice has two forms: social watching and individual watching. Social watching is relatively well known at the Manor. It occurs when patients or residents gather together in public places such as lounges, the nurses' station, or on the benches outside the Manor's entrance. Once gathered, participants may focus their attention on certain objects or events and consider them in some way.

One of the favorite pastimes of gatherings on patient floors is watching cars. This is more a patient than a resident practice. The former are less ambulatory and are more limited to the confines of their floors when they "sit around." They construct their sitting practices within these general limits. Watching cars in a group is something that patients can do on their floors with no physical effort beyond wheeling down to the lounge.

Watching cars is not usually a haphazard affair. Those who indulge in the practice may make it quite systematic. This involves "spotting" and counting the number of automobiles of a certain color or style. Those gathered compete to see who will first "spot" the specific feature of concern. They comment on the variety or popularity of this feature and often relate this to what "you used to see a few years back."

Vehicular events also are watched and evaluated. Typically, episodes of vehicular-event-watching begin when a participant indicates that someone in a specific car, bus, or truck is, for example, driving too close to the vehicle in front or too fast. Others turn their attention to the vehicle. A conversation then ensues that often generates a near life history of the driver that "shows why" he's driving the way he is. Episodes end with statements about "what they should do with people who drive like that."

Episodes may be embellished by a variety of conditions. When it is raining or snowing, weather often enters into the explanations for drivers' actions or statements about "what should be done." When the driver himself is visible, features of his appearance may become part of participants' explanation of his driving methods. For example, should it be discovered that a woman has done some particularly "bad" driving, an explanation already generated for it may be reconstructed to align it with the allegedly well known theory that driving behavior is sex-linked.

Patients who watch cars to pass time also keep track of staff vehicles in the employees' parking lot, which is visible from the south lounges on each floor of the Manor. Participants know which car belongs to which employee, if he drives more than one car, when he usually arrives at the Manor, where he usually parks, his routine in parking and leaving his automobile, who accompanies him, and the direction he comes from and departs to. When any of these things is mentioned by participants while chatting with "watched" employees, the latter occasionally wonder publicly how patients know "all that."

To those who engage in it, watching is serious business. Its significance is understandable in the context of the lives of those whose business at the Manor is largely passing time. After all, business is business, whether it is passing bad checks, celebrating the Mass, collecting garbage, or sitting around.

Take the following example of serious watching. Several patients are gathered in the south lounge on the third floor. Conversation is not focused on anything in particular. It drifts from the state of the weather to each patient's aches and pains. One patient, Lillian Koepke, points across the street to what she believes is a dog lying on the grass next to the curb. They all turn and look. Laura Kowalski, another patient, laughs and answers that what Lillian sees is a branch. Lillian insists that it's a dog and, specifically, a cocker spaniel. This leads to an amusing argument, full of laughter, scoffing, insistence, and joviality.

Two aides enter the lounge. Laura asks them what they see across the street. They both look and say it's some kind of broken barrel. The other patients present join the argument. All tease Lillian, who insists, "Just go out and pull the branches off, then, and you'll see that it's a dog!" They all laugh again.

Conversation shifts to other events out-of-doors for a while. Suddenly, Lillian informs everyone that she saw the dog moving. Laura and the rest look. Laura then says, "Now don't talk like that again. You know there's no dog there." No one is laughing now. Lillian is becoming angry. She turns to Connie, another patient, and states, "They're trying to make a regular liar out of me." Connie, who just entered the lounge and heard the very end of the argument, asks about the dog. Laura turns to her and flatly blurts, "Forget it, Connie. Just forget it!"

For the next few days, watchers in the south lounge are divided into two factions: those who are sympathetic to Lillian's claims about the dog and her feelings at being called a liar, and those who are "fed up because she's carrying a joke too far." Each faction castigates the other's credibility. Both are sarcastic. For example, Laura enters the lounge the next day and, in front of members of the other faction, jokes with Thelma Moser, "Is that dog still there?" Thelma answers snidely, "He sure is a nice dog. He stays put right there." Members of each faction accuse Lillian and Laura of "losing their marbles." Appeals are made to select members of the floor staff for support.

Floor staff, meanwhile, thinks "this is all just plain silly." Aides comment on "how ridiculous" a few of the patients are being. They also are irritated that the "dog crap has agitated them so much that some of them are making trouble for us by not wanting to sit at the same table [in the dining room]."

Finally, the object of controversy is removed. Factions continue to quarrel for a while. Members of each faction claim they were right. After five days, watching in the south lounge becomes more solidified. Avoidance subsides. Watching turns to other events. Conversation is friendly. Everyone has his marbles again.

Considerable social watching on patient floors is done at the nurses' station. Patients gather here in two ways. Some are wheeled and placed there by aides who "want to keep our eye on them." Others ask aides to wheel and place them there "alongside the other ladies." Station watchers typically are wheelchair patients. It is commonly believed that "if you're going to be anywhere outside your room, it might as well be the lounge or desk."

The dining room is considered dull and tiring by many patients. The lounge and station are felt to be "where all the action is."

Interaction between station watchers is quieter and less intensive than among lounge watchers. What station watchers look at is within easy hearing distance. When they comment about events involving floor staff and others at the station, they usually lean over and whisper. Sometimes those commented upon overhear them; sometimes they don't. In either case, they mostly ignore it as the idle talk of patients and go about their business.

Station watching is quite profitable for obtaining information and news about the daily lives of other patients and the work and private lives of staff on the floor. Watchers overhear a variety of things: other patients' requests; visitors' talk with floor nurses about the Manor and its clientele; floor staff conversations and their inside dope; and the nurses' side of telephone calls to and from relatives, physicians, morticians, top staff, the pharmacist, and unofficial parties such as boyfriends and spouses. Station watchers listen eagerly yet quietly. For the most part, floor staff carries on its business and talk as if they weren't present.

Another form of watching is done individually, mostly by bedridden patients. From their beds, they can see little that moves except what is in the hallway. By keeping track of what they see and hear through their open doors, they pass time.

Like watching cars out-of-doors, watching the hallway may be systematized. Some bedridden patients keep detailed accounts of the number of times other patients, often known to them by appearance only, walk by their doors. Some keep track of the relative rush of floor nurses and aides. And still others store mental notes on the number of "strange faces" that go by from day to day. While sitting with such patients, it is not unusual for them to gesture toward and comment on some passer-by in the following ways: "See that man? That's the sixth time he's walked by here this morning. I don't think he goes very far each time." "Just look at her. She's always in a rush. I don't think I've seen her *walk* by for a couple days." "I don't know who he is, but he walks by every morning and says, 'Good morning.' He's a nice man." "I think she must really stink. I've never seen her go by except in that striped dress."

Bedridden hallway watchers, like most people, try to make reasonable sense of their lives and what goes on around them. At the Manor, they do so in the context of their rooms and what passes their doors. A doorway offers a very narrow view of the local world to such watchers, who have access to little other information about everyday life in the home. And it is easy for them to generate fantastic explanations for its events. This is at least part of the reason such watchers sometimes "make no sense" to aides who occasionally talk with them about "this and that" at the Manor.

Talking

When patients and residents gather to talk but not necessarily to watch, they have favorite topics of conversation that reflect the features of their everyday lives: the Manor and its staff, reminiscences, the ongoing lives of their children and grandchildren, food, and their current aches and pains.

Gossip about the Manor ranges from talk about what is known of its financial status to recollections of former employees. As stories are passed from one person to another, those stories that may have some credibility are embellished in one way or another.

For about two weeks one summer, both patients and residents talked incessantly about the possibility that the Manor was being sold to a Lutheran organization. The gossip began one afternoon when Katy Miles was sitting on an outdoor bench "getting some air." A man who had been visiting a relative was leaving the building. On the way out, he joked briefly with Katy about the Manor. Although they were unacquainted, it is not unusual for departing visitors to stop momentarily and "chat with the poor old people."

The chat mostly focused on "how nice a place this is for all of you." Several of its amenities were mentioned, one of which was that it was "a great service that the Sisters [on the Manor's board] are doing for older people." As the man left, he jokingly said, "Let's hope that they don't sell the place to the Lutherans."

On returning to her room, Katy asked her roommate, Joan Borden, what she knew about the place being sold to the Lutherans. Joan said that she knew nothing but resolved to "find out about it." She is well known at the Manor for her ability to saturate a floor with news almost as fast as the public address system. Joan's attempts to "find out about it" turned out to be closer to a chain of announcements, for she asked others, "Do you know that I heard that this place might be sold to the Lutherans?"

The story spread fast. Its credibility was strengthened along the way with comments that it might be true since the "place is having financial problems anyway," and since Joan passed on the "fact" that a well-dressed, professional-looking man told Katy about it. This is what Katy had related initially to Joan. Clientele on all floors soon learned of the rumor. It was passed around in two ways. Interfloor acquaintances who gather on outdoor benches and in other public places at the Manor spread it between floors. Loud talk in such public places as lounges and the dining rooms spread it within each floor. Finally, members of the top staff heard of it when, over a week later, two enterprising residents decided to ask one of them about it. They were flatly reassured that there was no truth to the gossip. This too spread quickly. A few days later, talk of the Manor being sold subsided.

Patients and residents also pass time talking about the staff. It is either positive or negative, depending on the circumstance at hand. For example, the same clientele may describe aides as "just plain bitches" in a gathering that is complaining about the "bad service we get"[1] or "how they treat us here," and as "nice, respectful girls" in the presence of others who are lauding or formally inquiring about the Manor. Each is taken as a natural, taken-for-granted thing to say when the mood is clearly antistaff or prostaff, or assumed to be one or the other.

As in other circumstances, patients and residents generate explanations for their judgments of specific members of the staff. These are used to support both negative and positive evaluations. For example, the only black participants in everyday life at the Manor are some aides, a number of housekeeping girls, and a few nurses. All clientele and top staff are white. When patients and residents talk about the quality of treatment they receive from aides, they frequently use racial explanations. When a black aide is believed to be especially considerate, she is said to be "a credit to her race," or "really nice even if she is colored," or "better to have around than most of these white nurses." When a black aide is considered cruel or disrespectful, her behavior may be explained as "typical of her people," or "you just can't build a good home on nigger help," or "inbred in those darkies."

Patients and residents talk about each other constantly. Some

---

[1] Patients and residents call "service" what staff calls "care" or "work." This is evidence of clientele's rational interest in themselves as persons separate from their "role" in the home as an organization.

of this revolves around how mentally competent or incompetent specific persons are considered to be. Among residents and members of alertness cliques, this talk typically takes on a "poor thing" flavor. They "feel sorry," as they say, for those "poor things" on the third and fourth floors. Among patients and a few residents, talk of incompetence is often quite open, sufficiently so that the person being discussed may be within hearing range. In the dining rooms and lounges, it is not unusual to hear loud comments and see obvious gestures by some clientele about others that are present.

Some talk between patients and residents about others takes the form of news. When any one of them reminisces about his past, talks about his children, or reports on what he did when he "stepped out," it quickly becomes grist for conversation. Through such reporting and communicating, clientele come to know each other's family lives in a fair amount of detail.

As is commonly noted at the Manor, one "funny but sometimes painful" way to pass time is talking about and dealing with aches and pains. Few greetings are completed without some question about such ailments as "your swollen legs," "coughing spells," or "hemorrhoids."

Like floor staff, patients and residents talk a great deal about bowels. Some are plagued by constipation, whereas others suffer from diarrhea. Talk of bowels is varied: vivid personal descriptions of color and texture related to others who are gathered together; requests and sometimes long-term pleas to floor staff for laxatives, suppositories, enemas, stool softeners, and antidiarrheal preparations; recollections of experiences in obtaining help with toileting; complaints about the allegedly disgusting habits of certain patients who "piddle in bed," "poop all over the floor," "crap in others' rooms," "pee in my toilet instead of their own," or "just don't keep themselves clean"; and moaning about being "all pent up today," "sore down there," and "so weak from being loose that I have to stay near my room all day." One patient described the general concern of all clientele with bowels in this way:

> I know it's funny sometimes when you think about all the talk that goes on here about it [bowels]. But ya talk and ache about your bowels all the time. I don't know why an eighty-two-year-old woman has to be bothered with bowels. I'm so packed, if I don't have a movement, I'll

blow up. I sit down and hit my stomach and it's hard. Ever since I came here, it's been bowel problems all the time—all that rice and noodles that we eat.

A few patients and residents at the Manor pass time in fairly unique ways: two garden; two or three tend the gift shop; one conducts the rosary and manages the altar in the chapel; two or three sew bibs in the recreation area for use on "feeder" patients.

CEREMONIALS

Ceremonials also pass time, but they differ from sitting around in two important ways. First, they are conducted officially by the staff. Although sitting around may involve nurses and aides, they don't conduct it. Ceremonials are conducted in the sense that staff schedules their occasions, announces their time, presides over ritual, and dismisses the participants. Second, participating patients and residents treat ceremonials as special events. This means that one's decorum at ceremonials is different from what it is while sitting around. Ceremonial decorum is more formal than usual. One "dresses" for ceremonials and generally looks "decent enough to show oneself in public."

Ceremonials include Sunday Mass, Sunday Protestant service, weekly rosary, bingo, card parties, slide shows and films, birthday parties, outdoor picnics, Grandparent's Day (relatives invited), field trips, concerts given at the Manor by various community groups, discussion groups (book reviews, current events, etc.), and holiday parties. Most ceremonials occur monthly; some are only seasonal. Altogether, patients and residents pass much less time in them than they do in sitting around.

The schedule of the Manor's ceremonial occasions—the "activity calendar"—is published monthly by the activity director. The name is significant for it coincides with top staff's tacit belief that clientele are "really active" only on these occasions. At other times, they are believed to be largely doing nothing. This causes several members of the top staff to agonize about "getting these poor people up and around and doing something." On the whole, however, the total effort devoted to "activities" remains fairly stable from month to month.

Attending ceremonials usually involves some personal preparation. Notwithstanding their awareness, for example, that they are going to spend only 20 minutes on the second floor with other patients and residents saying the rosary, "getting ready" is important to participants. For most, this means donning one's Sunday best or at least "nicer things than usual." Men are likely to appear in suits and ties. Women typically put on more make-up than usual, wear a variety of bangles, cosmetics, and "dressy" dresses, and often carry small purses. Even the patient who ordinarily appears in bedclothes most of the day tries to look presentable in public. This seems momentarily odd, since on most occasions participants appear in what an aide once called "nursing home casual."

At ceremonies, residents mostly sit with other residents and patients with patients. The exceptions to this are products of inter-floor linkages between patients and residents. Furthermore, residents and patients each divide themselves along clique lines. For example, the Doherty group sits together at birthday parties and bingo. The smokers sit separately. Patient alertness cliques gather together and keep their distance from those who are considered to be "lacking in marbles."

Occasionally, as participants gather at ceremonial events, the segregation among clientele is violated. For example, in taking various wheelchair patients to birthday parties, aides rush up to the fifth floor and put them any place convenient to themselves. As one resident complained, "They just plunk those senile ones down anywhere." Many participants resent this practice, for it spoils what they believe to be their own proper dignity. When the occasion is not as solemn as a Mass or the rosary, such practices lead to considerable grumbling. At some parties, I have seen "senile" patients mercilessly gossiped about and antagonized throughout the event because they violate the "private" places of participants who believe themselves to be "above them." On such occasions, those "above" may even make a variety of obvious gestures that signify their feelings of having been physically polluted. They may wince at the sight of a violator or quickly turn away from him in a grossly arrogant fashion.

Solemn ceremonials include religious services and saying of the rosary. Clientele are quite respectful of the Manor's religious services. Regular churchgoers who cannot attend because they are ill or because the aides have not taken them to the chapel may become rather depressed. During solemn ceremonies, participants are decorous and solicitous of each other. Residents, for example, are unusually helpful toward those patients from whom, in other circumstances, they would cringe. Although patients and residents segregate themselves on solemn as on other ceremonial occasions, place violations are tolerated better on solemn ones. Any negative talk or gossip about place violations occurs well after the event rather than during it.

Leisure ceremonials such as parties and bingo games are not as universally respected as are solemn ones. Men are more likely to ridicule them than women. Some consider them "silly," "a bunch of old ladies playing kid's games," and "a lot of ladies talking about their aches and pains." Others simply feel that birthday parties and outings are just not for men. One of the enduring problems that some members of the top staff say they have is getting the men to come to these events.

THERAPY

Therapy is similar to ceremonials in that it is officially staff-conducted. It differs from them partly because it is not treated by clientele as a special, formal occasion. In going to therapy, patients and residents do not concern themselves with public presentability. They are more likely to appear in "nursing home casual" on therapeutic occasions than on ceremonial ones. Therapy also differs from ceremonials in that top staff defines it as rehabilitation and not simply recreation. Clientele, however, by no means feel this way about all forms of therapy at the Manor.

The various kinds of therapy include occupational therapy (OT), which may be diversional (crafts, painting, etc.) or functional (range of motion exercises, sanding); physical therapy (PT); group therapy, consisting of discussion sessions that the social worker conducts with residents; and reality orientation (RO), a drill-like procedure that presumably teaches time and place to "disoriented" patients.[2]

Patients and residents who participate in occupational, physical, and group therapies do so willingly, for the most part, but they participate in each for different reasons. Those who engage in functional OT and PT say that they "are helping ourselves get

[2] For discussions of the history and therapeutic rationale of RO, see James C. Folsom, "Reality Orientation for the Elderly Mental Patient," *Journal of Geriatric Psychiatry* 1 (1968): 291–307; and APA Hospital and Community Psychiatry Service, *Reality Orientation* (Washington, D.C.: American Psychiatric Association, 1969).

better." Their belief about what goes on in therapy approximates that of the staff members who conduct it. Clientele who participate in diversional OT and group therapy do not have a therapeutic view of what occurs in them. Although staff talks about them as therapeutic, clientele consider them to be "nice places to just kinda quietly sit around and be neighborly." Both resemble a coffee klatsch. The mood is cordial and leisurely; it is time for exchanging stories and gossip, usually without "annoying patients" around. Like leisure ceremonials, diversional OT and group therapy are attended mostly by women. Men believe them to be "women's stuff."

Reality orientation is for patients only. Moreover, it is for those whom top staff considers to be disoriented—that is, patients who are judged unable to keep track of time and place. Participating patients view RO in various ways. Some feel it is "a waste of time and just plain stupid." Some think it's "something to do to pass the time." A few say it's "like going to school." For the most part, participants do not believe RO is therapeutic. Patients who attend do so less willingly than clientele who participate in other forms of therapy. As one said: "They just swoop you up and bring you down here to play school. It's just plain stupid as far as I'm concerned. There's not much you can do about it except get mad."

Floor staff conducts RO. Its attitude toward it is similar to that of many participants but for different reasons. Both participants and floor staff believe RO to be "a waste of time" or at least "just a silly way to pass time," but floor staff believes it to be so because it disrupts its bed-and-body routines and, according to aides and nurses on the floors, "does absolutely nothing for the patient anyway." An aide put it this way:

> They [RO sessions] don't do nothing. You wheel 'em down there at eleven o'clock and that's one of the busiest times too. You've got baths to do and getting the patients into the dining room. What they [top staff] should do is just let us go and talk to the patients in the afternoon when things are quieter. But they don't allow that. I like to do my job but that reality thing is for the birds. I'm just not cut out for that stuff. Pam [aide who also conducts RO] is really getting fed up going up there everyday and saying, [mockingly] "Where do you live? What day is it?" and all that.

And an LPN:

> It's a waste of time. Why not leave them in their own
> little worlds? They're happy. So leave them be.

Before RO begins, patients and aides must gather themselves
and proceed to the particular place where it usually is conducted.
This is not *just* a matter of aides bringing patients to RO. A certain amount of negotiation is involved as well. For one reason
or another, some or all patients officially assigned to RO may not
want to participate in it. Likewise, aides who conduct it are
generally less enthusiastic about it than are their superiors. Participants, then, must take their proper roles and places before
therapy begins.

On occasion, a patient refuses to attend unless something he
wants is obtained for him. For example, a patient may threaten
not to cooperate (i.e., be a patient) unless an aide gets him a
few cigarettes. Or an aide may "make a deal" with a patient: if
he will come to therapy (and be a patient), "I won't bother you
too much with questions this time." Or an aide may plead with
a patient to behave (i.e., act like a patient), come along, and at
least sit quietly, or "I'll catch hell from upstairs." When the patient doesn't show some cooperation, the aide may invoke the
loss of her job.

Like patients, aides also either play their roles as therapists or
dismiss them (and RO), all with proper accounts, depending on
their felt needs at the moment.[3] When they decide to stage
therapy, aides may claim a variety of reasons for doing so: "It's
my job. Isn't it?" or "Who knows? It helps some of them sometimes," or (in reference to a superior whom they admire) "You
just hate to let her down, don't ya?" When they dismiss it, they
also account for their actions: "We're too busy for that reality
crap!" or "Look! Those who's alert is alert anyway and the senile
ones stay senile regardless of RO."

When the scene is set so that all participants have taken their
proper places and have at least tacitly decided to play their
respective roles as therapist and disoriented patients, RO begins.
RO sessions involve an aide as instructor and usually five patients

---

[3] See Marvin B. Scott and Stanford M. Lyman, "Accounts," *American
Sociological Review* 33 (1968): 46–62.

as students. Instructional materials, which are provided by top
staff nurses, consist of a chart (reality board) that lists the name
of the nursing home, its location, the date, the day of the week,
and the state of the weather, and a cardboard clock to teach
timekeeping. A typical session consists of drills by an aide. Patients are asked to read the items on the chart, one by one, and
then are quizzed on the content. The instructor next sets the
clock to official times of the day when patients are awakened,
fed, brought to RO sessions, and put to bed, and each patient
is asked what happens at those particular times. Correct (board-
oriented) answers to questions presumably mean that patients
are "oriented" and "accepting reality." At least, this is what top
staff believes.

The following exchange between an aide conducting RO and
a patient being asked about the state of the weather shows how
critical "place orientation" is in defining realism.

> AIDE: [Pointing to the weather on the RO board, which
> reads "raining."] What's the weather like today, Emma?
> *Emma turns her head slightly and quickly looks
> out the window.*
> EMMA: Well, it looks like the sun is shining kinda
> bright.
> *The sun happens to be shining at the moment.*
> AIDE: Are you sure? It says it's raining. Doesn't it?
> [Finger still pointing to board.]
> EMMA: Well, it doesn't look like it from here
> AIDE: What does it say here, Emma? [Directing
> Emma's attention to the board.]
> EMMA: It says it's raining.
> AIDE: [Warmly] That's correct. Very good.

And this exchange between an aide and another patient, Frank
Lueschen:

> *Aide points toward the board so as to direct all
> patients' attention there. From the patients'
> perspective, the aide appears to be pointing*

> *specifically to the line indicating the name of the home.*

AIDE: Can you tell me what day it is today, Frank?

FRANK: Murray Manor.

AIDE: No. What *day* is today? Look at the board again.

FRANK: It says Murray Manor.

> *The aide then drills the patients on board weather, but in quizzing them she frames her questions in a way that suggests they look outdoors for an answer.*

AIDE: Did you check to see if the weather is sunny today?

> *This directs patients' attention outdoors. The aide then addresses Frank but faces the board herself.*

AIDE: What's the weather like today, Frank?

FRANK: It's cloudy. Isn't it?

AIDE: No. It's sunny. See here, Frank. [Points to board.] *It-is-sunny.*

FRANK: It says sunny.

RO therapists do not formally distinguish between the "wrong" answers patients give. They treat all of them as mistakes and signs of confusion. However, not all "wrong" answers are mistakes by patients. On occasion, when they feel unduly put upon, they deliberately respond to RO items in a "confused" fashion.

> *Cyrus Cooper, a patient, has been wheeled to RO despite his request for a smoke beforehand. He grows irritated as the RO session proceeds and his desire for a cigarette increases.*

AIDE: [To Cyrus] Cy. What is the weather today?

CYRUS: I don't know.

AIDE: Try a bit harder, Cy. What is the weather today?

CYRUS: I don't know unless I get a cigarette!

AIDE: What place do you live, Cy?

CYRUS: I don't live any place.

Another part of RO is teaching timekeeping. As before, patients are tested for "realism" according to whether or not they answer questions in proper clock-oriented terms.

> *After drilling RO patients on the time they presumably are put to bed, an aide asks Agnes a question.*

AIDE: Now, Agnes. What time do we go to sleep at Murray Manor?

> *Patients were drilled that 8 o'clock is bedtime, but the mood of the session now is conversational.*

AGNES: Oh, that depends. Sometimes I go to bed at six and sometimes at nine. It depends on how busy I am and how tired.

AIDE: But you usually go to bed at eight. Don't you, Agnes?

AGNES: Well, sometimes, but not always.

AIDE: Yes, but we do go to bed at eight. Look here, Agnes. What does the clock say?

> *The clock is set for eight.*

AGNES: It says 8 o'clock.

AIDE: Yes. That's right. [Aide turns to the other patients.] We go to bed at eight at Murray Manor.

> *While pointing to the clock, the aide then asks each of the other patients what time he goes to bed at night.*

On occasion, patients answer an aide's questions drolly. The aide may laugh, often surreptitiously, but still insists on a "realistic" response. For example:

AIDE: Mazie. What do you do at 8 o'clock in the morning?

> *Mazie looks puzzled and stares around the premises.*

MARY [another patient]: [Shouting]   Get up and go pee!

> *The aide can't control her laughter, hides her face behind the clock, and chuckles. The mood of*

*the RO session is now definitely jovial, each
patient trying to outdo everyone else.*

AIDE: What did you have for breakfast this morning?

SOPHIE: We had eggs that were so hard that they're
like crackers. Crunch. Crunch. Crunch.

*One patient remarks that she can't remember what
she had for breakfast and another remarks . . .*

JOHN: [Sarcastically] She peed too hard and she can't
remember!

The world of time being taught in RO sessions to "orient patients to reality" is a strange one when compared to the practical world of time on the floors. On the floor, nurses and aides define clientele as "disoriented" and "confused" or not by the standards of normal work routine. What are considered to be disoriented statements in RO sessions are largely ignored on the floors. Should a patient mention that the day is Sunday when it is Wednesday, he'd officially be confused if he were in an RO session, but he'd not usually be labeled or treated (i.e., routinized as an annoyance) as disoriented if he were on the floor.

The reason that some patients do not keep track of time on the floor is not that they cannot. It is that it does not seem reasonable for them to do so. When it is reasonable, they become time-oriented. For example, one woman who is a regular participant in RO is rarely correct when she is quizzed in RO about the official time of various events in a "typical" day at the Manor. To her, "all of this is crazy." She usually is judged to be disoriented. One day, as she was trudging past the nurses' station, I asked her (with a mild sense of urgency) if she happened to know the time. She immediately looked at the clock above the station and said it was ten minutes past two. She was correct.

CONCLUSION

Clientele timekeeping on the floors of the Manor (and perhaps in most geriatric nursing homes) is not simply a matter of "putting in time" as in some hospitals nor of marking time while awaiting death as on "death row" in prison. Although death may be clearly in the air at the Manor, daily time on the floors is *passed*, which means that it is time itself and filling it that clientele are concerned with, not the time to mark (or put in) *toward* some fairly well delineated end (such as release from a hospital). A central issue of time for Manor clientele is how to fill it. In this chapter, I have tried to document the ways this is accomplished.

Throughout this book, I have taken the point of view that the events in social life are made by the people involved, and that what they accomplish depends greatly on place. At the Manor, people do not always consider the place at hand to be the floor, for example. In places other than the floor, their sense of time may be properly different than on it. The Manor's clientele live in multiple social worlds of time. To describe time as simply chronological or as simply "passing" would fail to do justice to the constructed, situated nature of time.

Dying and Death

Unlike patients' concern with watching automobiles or top staff's attempt to write total care plans, dying and death are commonly recognized occasions considered characteristic of the Manor's setting by all its participants. However, all do not consider them in the same way. Although all may be able to talk "casually" about them together and separately, not all talk is tacitly grounded in the same assumptions. Three worlds of dying and death exist in the home, adhered to separately by top staff, floor staff, and clientele. When the participants of one world deal with the participants of another, they may make trouble for each other.

EXPERIENCING VERSUS WITNESSING

When dying or death occurs at the Manor, it is clientele who physically *experience* them. Every day, patients and residents live with the knowledge that dying and death are imminent events for them. Not only do they experience dying and death themselves, but each one is also a *witness* to the experiences of others. If he is not seriously experiencing or witnessing, he still sees what he easily might become by observing those around him who are dying or dead.

Patients and residents differ somewhat as far as the continuity of their experiences with dying is concerned. When elders are admitted to the Manor as patients or become patients after entering as residents, staff considers them to be showing "obvious" signs of potentially dying. Both staff and clientele believe all residents and patients to be terminal in that they are aged, reside in the home, and are not fully expected to return to society "out there." Patients, however, are more likely than residents to show either certain "pointable" signs of dying (e.g., being completely bedridden, moaning, being emaciated, visibly decaying, or being virtually unintelligible) or to be defined by staff and clientele as soon to acquire these signs. Residents experience only periodic episodes of dying. Some have occasional epileptic seizures. Others have mild heart attacks or chest pains. Most take medications for nondisabling but chronic illnesses.

Patients and residents all define their futures in terms of death. In that respect, they all believe they are dying. Only the actual time of death is unknown. Take the following typical comments about their futures:

> *Gus Marsh [resident]:* My future, hell! What future is there for me? Blink! I'm the last of my family. No one's got a future here.
>
> *Homer Wilson [resident]:* At eighty-six? All I can think about is that God will call me someday. They'll take me out and bury me. I don't think about nothin'. I take it day by day. I don't plan on anything, because generally when you plan on somethin', it never turns out that way anyway. So I don't try to think or make any plans whatsoever. I take it day by day and leave the rest in God's hands.
>
> *Pearl Smith [resident]:* Well, I tell you. I take a day at a time. And you don't plan what might transpire because you just know it may all end anytime. So I might as well adjust myself and be happy and go along day by day.
>
> *Joan Borden [resident]:* I don't know. Well, if it comes,

it comes. If it comes tomorrow, it comes. It's coming for all of us anyway, sooner than later. No, it's no use to think about my future. It's settled! I wanna make use of my money first. I don't leave any money for anybody else. That's all I worked for—what I got.

John Varady [resident]: Lots of time, in my mind, I say it be better if I die. I got in Calvary cemetery—I got lot there and stone and everything. Lots of time I think, "Let me out, quick so I can go." What use we all here? We all going soon.

Katy Miles [resident]: I don't worry about it, if that's what you mean. I know just about what will happen, where I'll be buried, and all. So I don't worry about it. I just don't wanna be laying around here for months. That's all. Well, I've got everything taken care of so that if anything happens to me, I'll be taken care of. I don't plan much no more. I don't think I can. Not at my age. I suppose age makes a person stop planning. I don't know. My legs aren't too good either that I can run around even if I could. I think there's a lot more places that I could go to and things, but I have arthritis.

Bernice Hogan [resident]: Could we go on? There's no future. I just as soon die. I just ask God to please take me home. What should I live for? I ain't got nothing to live for. Kids don't come to see you. We're all sick here and upstairs they're worse. All we have left to look forward to is the end.

Elizabeth Tanner [patient]: There is no future for me. That's gone. I have nowhere to turn. What would I look forward to? Just sitting here? There's no future in that. I just feel hopeless. I did make plans at first, but none now. I just let Mother Nature take its course, I guess.

Bertha Thomas [patient]: I have no future. Tell me, when you're eighty-five, what are you going to do? There is no life here. If I could walk better . . . if it wasn't for that, I would call one of my friends, an attorney, and say, "You tell my daughter you wanna get me out of here." No. I would welcome, and I mean *welcome* if I could go to sleep. How do you like that? I hope I die. My minister gets mad. I say, "Please, please pray that I should die. I don't wanna live." I have nothing to stay for.

Laura Kowalski [patient]: No future. Not now anymore. I used to have a future before I got here. Nothing in particular but I did love my home. I used to plan a lot what I would like to do, see the grandchildren. You know, stuff like that. But not now. I don't know. I just feel that I'm stuck here and that . . . [weeps] I don't know what the future looks like. I don't know.

Stella Imogene [patient]: What kind of future could I think about? I don't make no plans because I can't walk around. See, it's a handicap for me. Now, I'm a person that lives day to day . . . ever since I was ill for so long, for so many years. They say the way my heart is, I could be dead tomorrow. See, when you have heart trouble, you don't know. People fall dead on the street and you never knew they were sick. That is the way I would like to. . . .

Betty White [patient]: I don't know. I can't see no future. When I get down in the dumps, I think I'm better off than some people. At least, I can wait on myself and I still have my mind. But it's hard to think that way. Well, I don't see no future . . . just death. That's all. Well, I don't know about death. It's a puzzle. Nobody's ever come back to tell us. I think I'm ready anytime.

Patients witness continuously what they define as vivid scenes of dying. Residents, on the other hand, witness what they believe is vivid dying on four occasions. First, when one of them experiences a physical crisis, such as a seizure or heart attack, other residents consider this to be an event when "he [or she] could have died."

Second, if the crisis is disabling to the degree that the person affected is believed to need skilled nursing care, he is transferred to the third or fourth floor and becomes a patient. To residents, a crisis that is followed by a "transfer upstairs" is considered evidence of "really dying." Such transfers are felt to be not only possible personal endings but also a social demise. As is often said after a resident witnesses a transfer that has followed a disabling crisis, "Poor thing. She's going and will probably never live a normal [first-floor] life again."

Third, several services at the Manor are located in places that make it necessary for those residents desiring to use them to observe dying patients. For example, the beauty and barber shop is located on the third floor. Also, many activities planned by the top staff include both patients and residents. This too provides residents with an opportunity to witness dying.

When residents enter the premises of those known to be dying, they are visibly wary. As soon as the elevator doors open onto a floor that houses dying patients, they give the premises much more careful scrutiny than is typical in other situations at the Manor. When the floor area immediately surrounding the elevator is believed to be adequately free from signs of dying, they proceed quickly to their destinations. Rarely do they continue to look about.

Fourth, two residents have wives on the third floor. Their daily reports to other residents on the health status of their spouses contribute to the vicarious witnessing of dying by those who listen. Another kind of vicarious witnessing occurs when residents inform others on the first floor of the status of friends whom they occasionally visit on the third and fourth floors.

Residents who have friends on patient floors try to avoid visiting them there. They sometimes go so far as to fetch patient friends from patient floors. When they can't do this, their visits on patient floors are notably short, infrequent, and uncomfortable. They sit in patients' rooms or lounges with obvious apprehension. When someone who shows what they consider to be signs of dying appears before them, they grimace or turn away.

Patients and residents differ in the extent to which each is likely to experience or witness death. Both believe that patients are more likely to die than residents. References are often made to the "fact that up there [or here], you're likely to go anytime." However, because they are ambulatory, residents are somewhat more likely to witness death than patients, and especially more than bedridden ones. In addition, when one resident hears about a death in the home, all are likely to know of it in short order. Among patients, there is a less comprehensive network of social contacts along which death news can spread. Although a few ambulatory patients may be witnesses to more deaths than any resident, residents as a whole hear of deaths or observe death clues more than patients do.

Bodies may be carried out of the building in two ways. Sometimes, especially at night, they are taken through the lobby and out the front entrance. This route is more visible to residents than to patients. More often. they are taken to the basement in the elevator and placed in an ambulance or hearse that has been parked at the rear of the building on the service ramp. When a body is released via the basement, both residents and patients whose rooms face the southeast or who sit and watch in the south lounge may witness death; in this case, see a body removed. This entrance is used mostly for deliveries of various goods, garbage pickups, and retrieval of bodies. If the first two are not occurring when vehicles park there, the third is likely to be.

Members of the floor staff do not die in the Manor. They are, however, more frequent witnesses of both dying and death than patients and residents. Not only does floor staff witness more dying and death, but it does so more intimately than either patients or residents, for the most part. For example, as an integral part of its routine work, floor staff handles and examines such evidence of dying as extreme emaciation and extensive physical decay. Clientele may observe these conditions, but they don't handle or treat them.

Floor staff is also a more intimate witness of dying and death than patients and residents in that it makes frequent and periodic inspection of dying patients in the course of bed-and-body work. It is witness to histories of dying. Because it observes dying and its symptoms over a period of time, floor staff is not as upset as clientele are when it encounters it. As one aide explained, "You get use to even the worst ones when you work around them a while."

In contrast to the floor staff, top staff does not witness dying and death to any great extent, nor does it extensively witness patient and resident responses to either. The witnessing of dying and death that top staff does primarily involves the administrator, administrative nurses, and the chaplain. Dying is witnessed indirectly by the administrative nurses in their periodic checks of routine floor work. They don't usually deal with the dying person nor with other patients' responses to dying per se. Rather, what they witness is only a by-product of their main concern with routine administrative work. What top staff sees of death is primarily an outcome of presiding over floor staff's work. A top staff nurse verifies a floor nurse's death diagnosis, calls the physician, and obtains a death pronouncement. If the administrator is in the building, he manages the death scene in terms of both space and timing: he sees to it that all floor personnel are properly involved and that clientele are kept distant; he may supervise the entire sequencing of events from death to removal of the body. The chaplain performs a variety of religious rituals depending, to some extent, upon the religious affiliation of the deceased.

Top staff's regular administrative work affects its witnessing of death and dying in two ways. First, dying is believed to be part of the routine work of floor personnel, not of top staff. Second, when top staff witnesses death, it is involved administratively, officially or unofficially. As one aide put it, "They do their bit and if the funeral men take too long to come, they leave."

DEATH WORLDS

Clientele and Death

Talk of dying is never completely separate from talk of death among patients and residents. Dying is suffering and, as they say, "Who wants to suffer!" To them, it is only "sensible" to want to be dead if one is suffering. As for the dead, they are believed to have finished with the "worry" that comes from having to "be a burden" on others. The following express their practical view of the intimate link between dying and death.

> Well, for her I was grateful [that she died]. 'Cause they said there was nothing to her. And I know she was a good person and if there was a heaven she would go there.
> _____
> Not that I like to hear of anybody dying, but as far as that [death] bothers one—no. We all have to go, and we don't know when. And she was ninety-three years old.
> _____
> As long as God leaves Mother [wife] here with me, I'll stay with Mother. When God calls her—which is a terrible thing to say—I hope it comes soon. When you know that she can't get well, it's pitiful to sit there and watch her. She's in pain most of the time . . . very severe dia-

betes. And I hope it's tonight. That's an awful thing to say. Awful. 'Cause I dearly love her.

I hope that I don't live to be too old. That's all. I mean I hate to be a burden or a worry all my life to someone. I have never been before. And then you wonder and just hope that when your time comes, you go quickly. That's all.

I took part in many informal conversations about dying and death at the Manor. On occasion, I deliberately tried to steer talk toward either dying or death alone, but I was rarely successful. In a gathering one time, a participant pointedly asked me, "How can you talk about one without the other? You tell me that." In another attempt, a man flatly stated, "When you're dying, you're dead. That's all there is to it."

When someone dies at the Manor, there is no general gloom among other patients and residents. As many suggest, death is a very reasonable thing to expect "in a place like this." When anyone hears of the death of someone he did not know well, he may be curious and politely sympathetic, but he is not especially mournful or depressed.

As patients and residents gather in the lounges or other public places, they exchange opinions about dying and death whenever one of them mentions that he "just happened to look in on" or "heard about" a dying person at the Manor. Typically, the ensuing exchange involves at least two kinds of statements. First, someone says that the suffering is "terribly depressing." Occasionally, another person adds that the dying person is "taking it very hard" or "taking it very well." Second, talk of death closes the conversation. This usually takes one of two forms, depending on whether discussion has turned to their own futures or is still oriented to the dying person. When it is centered on their own futures, comments are made about the personal desirability of death should one begin "really suffering" [dying]. Everyone agrees. When it is still oriented to the dying person, it is likely to be said that "death would be a blessing for him" or "I hope she passes for her sake, the poor thing."

On occasion, a person who is quite visibly dying appears or is pushed into the company of a group of residents or "alert" patients. When this occurs, the group becomes increasingly irritated the longer the intruder remains with them. It is not uncommon for the "alerts" to look away or to show both consternation and anxiety. Their comments also make it obvious that they are persons "rudely" being subjected to the frightening symptoms of dying, "without any regard for *our* feelings."

In such "uncalled for" circumstances, talk of dying is exasperated but whispered. Anyone may lean over to another and complain, "They shouldn't bring people who are that bad in here!" "It's best to keep those poor people separated." When such an intrusion occurred in his area of the dining room, one patient, who later claimed to have lost his appetite, whispered through clenched teeth: "See that man. He must be suffering. I'd rather be dead than that way. How can anyone eat with that around?"

Patients and residents claim to "feel sorry" for the dying—to them, a proper sentiment to express—but this does not mean that they are willing to personally indulge them. They "feel sorry" at a distance. For example, residents are usually quite willing to talk about "visitation programs" to the sick, and they may complain among themselves or to the activity director about the "need" for scheduled visits. This usually is punctuated with talk of "Christian duty," "those poor people suffering alone," and "everyone wanting a visitor or a kind voice in time of need." But whenever visitation is scheduled, residents typically are reluctant to engage in it. As they say, "I just don't have time today," or "I've just been so tired lately that I better not," or "I'm expecting a visitor this afternoon." Others groan or simply "forget."

When dying patients talk of dying, they express an urgent desire for death. Some say that it is unfortunate that one has to suffer so before he "passes." Others complain that it is the waiting that is so agonizing. Three of them put it this way:

Why do we have to suffer? That's the thing. God help us. I wish it would come soon. Let it end. When? When?

Who likes life, anyhow? Well, it's just that I wanna pass away. That's the one. I wanna pass away. That's it. Well, what should I do? The rest of the afternoon I don't know what I'm gonna do. God help me. I wanna go. I'd like to pass away. It would be quiet and nice.

I'm bad and they're [other dying patients] worse yet. So why a person has to live that kind of life? If you're old, you should die and be done with. They're no good to nobody. They're just like a vegetable. I hope someday I go to sleep and I don't get up. I only ask God to give me peace as soon as possible. Take me out of this world.

Clientele are rather perfunctory in referring to death. Dying patients matter of factly describe the characteristics of death as opposite to what they consider the most prominent features of dying. If dying for them means pain, death is blissful relief. If dying means being annoyed by others' complaints of the burden involved, death means quiet solitude. Residents and patients who are not dying describe the character of death in a simpler fashion than do visibly dying patients. Since dying, for them, means chronic dependence, death is simply the "end of useless living," of "being a burden."

The one exception to this occurs when patients and residents talk about a close or intimate friend who has died. Friendship makes death an interpersonal ending in addition to a public one at the Manor. When a patient's or resident's close friend dies, he usually refers to the death mournfully. The deceased is missed. Occasionally, those who survive the friendship are in despair at the loss. A resident recalls her friend in this way:

> There's one that died from this floor. She came the same day I did. She was Miss Custer. She'd never been married. She was a schoolteacher. She was a very nice person, and real friendly. I miss her. I'm really sorry that she's gone. She was as lonesome as I was. I was alone. So we used to visit each other. Yes, I liked her very much. I felt awful bad when she died.

And a male patient, when asked about being depressed by news of a death at the Manor, said:

> Oh, not unless he's a personal friend. Otherwise, I don't give a damn. Of course, I feel it because I know it's a life, but it doesn't affect you that much. Now George [roommate who's his friend] . . . if there's anything wrong with George, I would feel sorry for him. I like George and I think he's a hell of a nice fella.

Floor Staff and Death

In working with patients and residents, floor staff takes account of what it believes is their relative alertness. To floor staff, being alert means that one has personal sensibilities about death. In the company of those considered alert, floor staff avoids making mention of anyone who has died. Among patients not considered alert, nurses and aides talk openly and audibly about death. The death talk is quite graphic and glib. For example, it is not unusual to hear aides shout to each other across a patient's room, asking if some recently dead person's body has been prepared yet. Typically, the responding aide lists any other things to be done if the body has been only partially readied. She may mention the need to change bedding due to the release of fecal waste or urine; washing the body; removing such personal belongings as glasses, rings, and watches; and removing dentures from the deceased's mouth.

On one occasion, an aide complained to another aide about the difficulty she had "getting her [the deceased's] dentures out of her mouth" as she was changing the bed of a patient not considered alert. The "unalert" occupant of the room was seated near the window, watching and listening as the aides chatted. The working aide explained the technique she used that "finally worked." It was a matter of "kinda grabbing her lips and cheeks and holding them tight as you reach under the gums and flip 'em out." As they walked out, one said to the other, "I'll have to try that one next time." The patient muttered under her breath, "What a thing to talk about."

Regardless of whether the patient or resident in their company is alert, aides readily converse about the bed-and-body work they have completed with the dying (as opposed to the dead) and what yet remains to be done. They ask each other to help with such tasks as lifting heavy patients, turning them for "open, ugly bedsores," and taking someone to toilet who's "so helpless, he'll 'go' any one of these days." Such talk is considered an everyday, practical part of routine work on the floors.

The openness of floor staff's death talk does not depend simply on what it considers differences in clientele sensibilities. It is indirectly linked to what staff believes to be the greater vulnerability of "alert" clientele. As one aide explained, "It's not good to talk about death in front of the more alert ones. If they got frightened, it would just make your work that much harder." Aides feel that if they take into consideration the differences in clientele sensibilities to death, routine work with them is likely to be smoother than if they don't. Floor staff's *conception* of "alert" patients' alleged possible reactions to death and the potential impact on normal work routine leads it to treat the topic of death differently in their presence than it does in the company of others. It is not floor staff's actual experiences with death-panicked, alert patients running amuck and disrupting normal routine that affects death talk, since alert patients don't panic at the news of death.

Floor staff's death world also is sensitive to top staff presence on the floors. One exception to top staff's usual absence from the floors occurs in the event of death. When someone dies, the administrator, top staff nurses, and the chaplain appear and preside over floor staff's death work. This alters floor staff's death work and talk. With top staff present, all clientele are treated as sensitive to the topic of death. Aides are careful to whisper death talk and to conceal bed-and-body work on the deceased from everyone.

Floor staff believes that its superiors "want everything hush-hush about the subject in front of any of the people [clientele] here." Both from the directives it receives from top staff members when deaths occur and from the behavior of top staff in death situations, floor staff feels that it is expected to act "different than usual" on such occasions. As an LPN on the fourth floor said:

> When someone dies, Miss Timmons calls up to get all the patients out of the halls and into their rooms. We're supposed to close all the doors. So everyone runs around getting patients into their rooms. Some of the patients get mad because they don't want to be shoved around. Of course, I have to do my job. Up here, I don't think that death frightens the other old people. I don't push my opinion too much because then they'd think I don't care about the other patients or that I was morbid.

Floor staff's "different" treatment of death when top staff is on the premises tends to disappear as the members of top staff leave the death scene. In a death situation where those present are "unalert" patients and floor and top staff personnel, there is a considerable amount of whispering in an atmosphere that is cautious and solemn. Whispering and solemnity do not result simply from top staff presence, but rather from its presence in a death scene. When top staff is on a floor at other times, there is an obvious increase in cautiousness, but there is no extensive whispering or solemnity. As soon as it is known that top staff has left, death talk and bed-and-body work on the deceased become clear and obvious.

Top Staff and Death

When top staff witnesses dying, it is a relatively momentary and residual aspect of its administrative work. When it witnesses death, top staff mostly presides over it. It appears on the floor and directs nurses and aides in the variety of tasks associated with preparing a deceased person in a nursing home for the mortician. Its presence on the floor involves a rather solemn performance. When it presides, all floor behavior (that of both clientele and floor staff) is scrutinized for decorum, solemnity, and quiet urgency. Floor staff is rather sensitive to this. It changes its definition of death from being a routine part of work to being something special.

At a death scene, top staff's talk with clientele contrasts dramatically with the standard glib form it takes in passing. It is highly clientele-oriented and manipulative. Any patients or residents encountered are indulged in conversation. For example, responses to clientele statements about their health are inquisitive and conciliatory. Top staff tries to keep the topic of death out of conversations. As a matter of fact, while such talk proceeds, top staff tends to lead clientele away from a death scene.

In a death scene, no matter how "unalert" someone usually is considered to be, top staff converses with him. This occurs even if top staff must supply the entire content of talk. Top staff doesn't talk of death in the presence of any patient or resident, "alert" or otherwise. This contrasts with floor staff's definition of death talk as routine and open in the presence of those whom it considers, as aides says, "out of it most of the time."

To top staff, the practical world of death is separate from the world of dying. Dying is considered to be a normal, taken-for-granted part of floor staff's work. When deaths occur, however, they are treated as special events. As a top staff member typically says of his work when he is informed of a death, "I'll put this to one side for a while." When the body of the deceased has been adequately prepared and the death scene properly staged, members of the top staff take leave with comments such as, "Well, I'll get back to work since everything up here is under control now."

Top staff's talk and behavior at a death scene differs from its talk away from it. When top staff expressly talks *about* dying and death, it doesn't separate the two. Both are said to be treated as "routine things" in the home. As the in-service director explained:

> That stuff of protecting the patient is a bunch of old horseshit. Patients don't react. When everyone starts running around closing doors, that's when they get an idea that something must have happened. The new idea is to just try and be as natural as possible. I feel that that's the best thing. A lot of hush-hush stuff about death is left over from hospitals. You know, in hospitals they close all the doors when someone dies. Well, hell! Everyone knows something's happened when you do that. I think it's stupid.

And the director of nursing:

> When someone dies, I used to try and protect the other patients. We'd clear the halls and hide the body from everyone. I never treated death as part of my work. Somehow, it was always something separate—something to deal with differently than the routine care of patients. It's the hospital idea. That's the practice in hospitals. I was afraid that patients would get frightened at death and panic. So we protected them.

Running through top staff's descriptions of how death allegedly is treated at the Manor are references to the current conception of death in the nursing profession. Top staff nurses cite examples from the geriatric and nursing journals to which they subscribe about the need to "treat death as a normal and routine part of health care." They mention various books which they have read, the most common of which is Elisabeth Kübler-Ross' *On Death and Dying* (1969), which advocates the normal and open treatment of dying and death. The assistant director of nursing compares current with older conceptions of death in the training of nurses:

> We used to take all kinds of precautions. We were told in nurse's training to hide the body, cover the dead, and to get everyone out of the hallways when they wheeled the body out. Nurses are not trained like that anymore. Now,

they're trained to just be natural and not get all frantic when someone dies.

It is evident that top staff's treatment of dying and death is one thing in the context of a death scene and another in situations where its members speak, as self-defined geriatric professionals, about the care of terminal patients. In the one instance, in its practical relations with staff and clientele on the floors, death is a special event separate from dying. In the other, its reading of professional literature informs it that these should not be separated in practice. Considering itself professional, top staff attempts, as far as possible, to use the language of *current* geriatric practice and to be informed of and offer "appropriate" opinions about *current* geriatric care.

DEATH NEWS

Whether news of death is welcome or not depends on one's point of view. Differences between clientele and top staff views of death suggest separate orientations to death news. Patients and residents are eager to be informed of deaths that occur in the home. Top staff tries to contain death news because, in practice, it believes such information is frightening to patients and residents. Floor staff works to support top staff's sentiments, partly because the latter is its superior and partly because floor staff believes that its routine work might be disrupted and made difficult otherwise.

Floor staff attempts to contain death news in a variety of ways. When floor personnel discover that a patient or resident might have died, they are officially required to page one of the top staff nurses immediately. The public address system is audible to everyone in the home simultaneously. When someone pages a top staff nurse because of a death, she never announces the purpose of the call. Rather, a top staff nurse is told to come to the specific floor where the death has occurred.

The manner in which pages for death confirmations are made contrasts with pages for other matters. Death pages are less casual than others. Also, they *command* the presence of a superior on the floor. Pages not related to deaths usually are made as requests. The differences serve as clues to death events. As a ward clerk explained: "I can always tell when something is wrong. They *tell*

Timmons or Singer to come to the third or fourth floor. When they say, 'Miss Timmons or Mrs. Singer, please call the third or fourth floor,' then you know that nothing is going on."

Not only do various floor and top staff members initially learn of possible deaths through "concealed" death pages, patients and residents do as well. Whenever a regular page is made over the public address system, patients and residents show little visible response and seldom make specific comments on it. However, when a page commands a top staff nurse (and sometimes the administrator) to come to a particular floor, it is not uncommon for patients and residents to react in one of two ways. They may look up from what they are doing and give obvious signs of listening further or scrutinizing their premises. Or they may ask themselves or someone near them, "I wonder what's happening?" Everyone is on the alert that, as one patient put it, "maybe something gives." This is the first stage in the spread of death news.[1]

Although processing death at the Manor officially requires only the presence of one top staff nurse, other top staff members hear the page to her, suspect a death, and converge on the death scene. If their suspicion is confirmed, they begin to preside over the event.

From the patients' and residents' point of view, it is extraordinary to find so much of the "top brass" around—"all those official-looking people." In routine, day-to-day work on the floors, they are rarely seen, especially the administrator, social worker, and chaplain. Moreover, top staff is not just passing by but is strangely indulgent of clientele as it keeps an eye on the death scene. To patients and residents, this too is rather unusual.

This is the second stage in the spread of death news. What was only a suspicion of some special event is now confirmed with the presence of special participants. Although patients or residents may not yet know definitely that a death has occurred, they are aware of the possibility. As they momentarily explain the presence of "top brass" and their solemnity: "I'll bet you someone had a stroke," or "Someone must have passed." The spread of death news

[1] This stage and the following ones occur when a death is discovered and concealed from clientele by members of the Manor's staff. The spread of death news skips stages when a death is discovered by clientele. For example, occasionally someone collapses and dies in a public place such as the hallway or dining room with patients or residents present. In such cases, death news is spread without page clues.

among patients and residents beyond this point is contingent on
social relations and physical arrangements in the home.

Staff takes advantage of a number of physical arrangements to
contain the spread of death news. Among these are closing doors,
pulling curtains, feigning routine patient treatment, and removing
a body while clientele are dining.

Take the business of hiding the body. Before a body is considered ready for the mortician, it is washed and wrapped. Top
staff considers this to be a morbid affair for other patients or
residents to witness or to be aware of. Ironically, it shows little
of the same concern that aides hide bed-and body work on the
dying, which may be more audible and vivid than work on the
dead.

Until recently, whenever someone died who shared a room with
another patient or resident, his body was removed discreetly to
an empty room, where the body was then prepared. When the
body was being moved, clientele standing or walking in the hallway in the immediate vicinity were calmly urged toward the other
end, and the fire doors were sometimes closed after them. But at
the present time, on the third floor, almost all rooms are filled to
capacity, so there are no empty rooms available to "hold the body"
or prepare it for the mortician. Staff has no private place to do its
body work in the usual perfunctory way.

Responding to this situation, top staff directs floor personnel to
take advantage of the "normal" appearance of bed-and-body work
by passing off the process of preparing the dead as treating the
seriously ill. It is routine for aides to enter patients' rooms and
give them bed baths. While doing so, they may pull the curtain
that separates patients sharing a single room. This normal routine
also allows them to process a dead body.

Aides wash the body of the deceased, as if they were performing the usual bed-and-body work on living bedfast patients. For
example, when an "alert" roommate is present on the other side of
a pulled curtain, aides preparing a body refrain from talking about
it in a depersonalized fashion, since this would signify to the roommate that it is lifeless. The dead patient is adjusted (face and
body posture) to make him appear to be sleeping. His eyes are
closed, his mouth shut, and his head turned to one side. The appearance of the "sleeping" dead and the sleeping living are strik-
ingly similar.

The security of using physical arrangements to support the living appearance of the dead may be as sound as the security of empty rooms in containing death news. But both have certain disadvantages that can threaten staff's attempt to prevent the living from becoming aware of the dead. When an empty room is used to prepare a body, staff does little or nothing to make the deceased look alive. Because of this, it is important to keep the door of such a room closed. This entails a certain amount of vigilance since clientele's doors have no locks; patients' doors, in contrast to residents', usually are open; and some patients habitually wander into various rooms to visit or simply "look around." When an occupied room is used to prepare a body, and then the body is left there, it becomes necessary to act as if the person were living. Any "slips" are potential clues to death.

Patients and residents also take advantage of physical arrangements, but to *obtain* death news. Some of them are "specialists" in that they have direct access to certain arrangements that present accurate death clues and make it their business to be the vigilant keepers of these clues. For example, a few patients and residents who have rooms that overlook the ambulance ramp at the rear of the building "keep an eye," as they say, on "what's going on out there." Others frequent different floors for a variety of reasons, such as visiting wives or friends or to obtain services. Such persons are strategic links in the diffusion of death news between floors. When such links weaken, death news is more easily contained on a floor.

Once a patient or resident on any floor knows that a death has occurred, there are certain places that make for its rapid diffusion throughout the Manor. These are places where gatherings occur, such as the dining room, the lounges, or the lobby. Death news is easily spread in these places as table conversation, idle talk, and chitchat.

One final and unequivocal source of death news is the obituary page published daily in local newspapers. If patients and residents do not already know of the death of someone at the Manor whom they knew by name, they are likely to know of it in a day or two. This is rare, though, since death news diffuses rapidly in the home.

To patients and residents, it is important that death news be accurate. As soon as they become aware of the death of an acquaintance, they "invest" themselves in socially closing off his life. This means two things. First, the deceased is recalled, and varied features of his known life in and out of the Manor become a major topic of the talk that passes time. What he was and the consequences of his death are speculated upon. The sentiments expressed clearly accentuate the positive. The deceased is eulogized to some extent despite the fact that he or she may not have had "all his marbles" when living. He is now believed to "finally be at peace." Many questions are mulled over and rehashed: "I wonder how his daughter feels?" "Do you think her husband will live much longer now that the wife is gone?" "Melba [deceased's roommate and close friend] will probably take it real hard. Do you think she'll get over it?" Second, closing off the life of an acquaintance entails not only a rearrangement of sentiments about the person but also public evidence that this is so. Sympathy cards are sent. Condolences may be expressed to relatives.

On one occasion, residents became quite angry at being the victims of a false rumor about one of them who had died while at a hospital. The rumor began when a resident, Millie Ransom, who has a telephone in her room, was urged to call the hospital one morning "to see how Velma is making out." When Millie finally called, she allegedly was told by a nurse at the hospital that Velma had died. Soon after, Millie walked to the receptionist's desk in the front lobby and related to Sister Marilyn what she thought she had been told on the telephone. Joan Borden (alias the "newspaper") overheard this and immediately rushed down the first-floor hallway, urgently informing all residents she passed of the news. She even told Velma's roommate and close friend, Dorothy Porath.

The news became the major topic of all talk on the floor. Dorothy Porath was quite distressed. Several residents tried to comfort her. Everyone acquainted with Velma began thinking about expressions of sympathy. A collection was begun to send flowers.

The next day, a resident encountering one of Velma's relatives in the lobby expressed her sympathy. The relative was surprised and told her that Velma, on the contrary, was doing quite well and would be back at the Manor in about ten days. News that the rumor had been false spread quickly. So did a number of accusations that Millie "is losing her marbles." The residents felt that they had been made fools of, personally and publicly.

Clientele appreciation of both death and definitive death news is not morbid or "abnormal." Like many aspects of living and dying in a place such as the Manor, it is quite reasonable when understood in the context of its contingencies. Clientele appreciation exists at two levels of their daily experiences. They are implicitly grateful for news of a death because sharing this news helps them to pass the time. As individuals, they say they will be grateful for death as a release from the repugnance of dying. It is important for death news to be accurate because, at either level—whether sharing death news or being personally grateful for death—appreciation involves the investment or expression of sentiment. Inaccuracy produces that "extra work" involved in reconstructing one's sentiments, such as rather abruptly changing the tone and mood of one's expressions about the "deceased." These may in turn necessitate explanation and justification.

CONCLUSION

In this chapter, I have tried to show how place influences the death worlds of the Manor's participants. Depending on place, these worlds remain fairly well-insulated from each other. For example, in places whose participants are limited to clientele, the death world involved allows the public appreciation of death to be a very reasonable thing. In other places, where participants are limited to top staff, the world at hand induces members to take for granted that, indeed, clientele may appreciate, or at least not respond negatively toward death. Comparing worlds of death in exclusive clientele places with those in exclusive top staff places would suggest a certain affinity to exist between them.

In certain other places at the Manor, death worlds virtually collide. This may seem rather strange when, in their separate places, they appeared so compatible. For example, the seeming compatibility of the worlds of top staff and clientele regarding clientele responses toward death "make trouble" for their respective participants when both are present in the place where a death has occurred. Thus, one cannot use features of the varied social worlds in separate places to predict the outcome of the encounters between these worlds in other places. Each place is likely to have its own social logic, which may or may not be consistent with that of another place.

Index

Age Studies